THE MEDICAL RISKS OF LIFE

Dr Stephen Lock is Editor of the *British Medical Journal*. He qualified as a doctor in 1953 and has held various hospital appointments, including that of a senior registrar in pathology at Lewisham Hospital. He obtained the M.R.C.P. in 1963 and was elected F.R.C.P. in 1974. He joined the *British Medical Journal* in 1964 and was Medical Correspondent for the B.B.C. Overseas Service from 1966 to 1974. His other publications include *An Introduction to Clinical Pathology* and *Health Centres and Group Practices*. He has also written articles on haematology and medical writing in British, American, Swiss and Finnish journals. Dr Lock is married and has two children.

Dr Tony Smith is Assistant Editor of the *British Medical Journal*. He qualified as a doctor in 1959 and after a series of hospital appointments became a full-time medical journalist in 1965. He is now Medical Correspondent for *The Times*, and has published two textbooks on family planning. Dr Smith is married and has three children.

Dr Stephen Lock and Dr Tony Smith are joint authors of *Better Medical Writing* (under the pseudonym of Charles Thorne) and were consulting editors of the *Reader's Digest Family Health Guide*.

The Medical Risks of Life

STEPHEN LOCK
and
TONY SMITH

PENGUIN BOOKS

Penguin Books Ltd, Harmondsworth, Middlesex, England
Penguin Books, 625 Madison Avenue, New York, New York 10022, U.S.A.
Penguin Books Australia Ltd, Ringwood, Victoria, Australia
Penguin Books Canada Ltd, 41 Steelcase Road West, Markham, Ontario, Canada
Penguin Books (N.Z.) Ltd, 182–190 Wairau Road, Auckland 10, New Zealand

—

First published 1976

—

Copyright © Stephen Lock and Tony Smith, 1976

—

Made and printed in Great Britain by
Cox & Wyman Ltd, London, Reading and Fakenham
Set in Intertype Baskerville

To our children
Adam, Caroline, Harriet, Imogen and Sebastian –
for whom the contents may matter

CONTENTS

INTRODUCTION

CHINESE mandarins, it is said, used to pay their physicians only so long as they remained well; as soon as any official fell ill all payment ceased. There is more wisdom in this approach than might at first appear. Until comparatively recently doctors could give sound advice on how to prevent much illness but could do little to cure it. Indeed, the sufferings of serious illness were often made worse by fashionable physicians – both Louis XIV and Charles II suffered torments on their deathbeds at their doctors' hands. A false impression has been given by the success of antibiotics and vaccines in eradicating the infectious diseases such as tuberculosis, syphilis, typhoid and smallpox. Though surgery, X-rays and drug treatment can now deal with some types of cancer with the same certainty that penicillin cures pneumonia, modern medical technology has no answer to the main, killing diseases of modern civilized man – coronary thrombosis, stroke and advanced cancer. The best it can offer is relief of symptoms and slowing of the natural progress of the disorder.

Infectious diseases were controlled medically only after the bacteria and viruses responsible had been identified and their behaviour largely understood. The same process is now under way with non-infectious diseases, though the identification of their causes is far less easy. Probably 80 per cent of cancers will eventually be found to be due to external factors such as diet, chemicals, atmospheric pollutants, drugs, tobacco and alcohol; at any rate that is the estimate of Sir Richard Doll, the Oxford professor of medicine who with Sir Austin Bradford Hill was responsible for proving the link between cigarette smoking and lung cancer. In heart disease and some forms of mental illness, heredity and personality may prove to be of greater importance, but even in these conditions environmental factors are known to exert powerful influences.

Within the last few years the study of these factors has developed into a new science. Departments of epidemiology, often linked with social medicine, have sprung up in university medical schools and almost every medical student is now taught something about the subject. Epidemiology is medical detective work. Starting with little more than the fact that a disease exists, the epidemiologist tries to identify every factor that might explain why it affects some people but not others. Sex, age, race, social class, occupation, climate, altitude, diet, hobbies – all these variables must be compared in those with the disease and those without it.

When epidemiological research is done carefully and unemotionally valuable information is often forthcoming, such as the identification in the winter of 1975 of a link between cancer of the uterus and hormone replacement therapy in menopausal women. Only too often, however, an association is spotted and given publicity before there has been time to investigate it fully. It is never easy to disentangle chance associations from those which lead to understanding of the cause of a disease. Accounts in the press and on television of newly discovered causes of cancer or coronary thrombosis have tended to devalue their significance in the eyes of the public; yet some of these connections are important. In this book we have tried to give an objective account of the established facts and current theories about the causes of illness, to describe the results of past changes in behaviour, and to forecast the effects of new social trends. The data presented should help to put the hazards into perspective – it is pointless someone getting excited about being poisoned by mercury in tuna fish while he is poisoning himself by smoking sixty cigarettes a day – but there is very little advice of the 'give up drinking or die' type.

In any case, large-scale advances in a nation's health depend as much on social changes brought about by the

State as on medical action by doctors. In the nineteenth century improvements in sewage and education did as much for health as all the many medical advances. Today the countries with the best health statistics are those which have abolished poverty – Switzerland, Norway, Sweden, Denmark and Finland. Too many of the population in Britain are still struggling with health hazards that ought to be extinct – smoke-laden air, decaying housing and dangerous industrial occupations. At the same time too many are dying from the diseases of affluence, the results of too much food, too much drink, too much tobacco and too little exercise. The relative importance of all these factors – and many others less known but also important – is the subject of this book.

Finally, we are indebted to many friends for their advice and help, but particularly Dr J. C. Petrie, who read through the whole manuscript, though responsibility for the statements contained in it is entirely ours. We owe a great debt to our two secretaries, Linda Beecham and Wendy Smart, for their heroism in typing, and retyping, the script, and to Adam Lock, who largely compiled the index.

STEPHEN LOCK

TONY SMITH

Chapter 1

LIFE PATTERNS

*'In this world nothing can be said to be certain,
except death and taxes'* – *Benjamin Franklin*

THROUGHOUT life outside circumstances have an important influence on health, starting at the earliest stage; conception. Boys seem more likely to be conceived early in the menstrual cycle than girls, which may be why male embryos more often miscarry. The age of the parents at conception and their social class also have important links with the risk of birth abnormalities and the baby's subsequent health (see p. 278), as may the area where the child subsequently lives. In England the gradient for both sickness and mortality rates gradually increases from the south east to the north west. These variations are linked with social and economic factors whose individual roles are difficult to disentangle – but one firm correlation is that the higher the sickness and death rates in a given population, the greater the proportion of occupied and retired people in social classes IV and V.

Although some people have put the blame purely on geographical factors, pointing out that the regions with high rates tend to be those with less favoured climates and which were not heavily populated before the Industrial Revolution, the Scandinavian countries (with their much less stratified societies) have a worse climate and yet considerably lower mortality rates. Even peoples living in apparently similar cultures show remarkable differences in their illness and death rates. Thus compared with the English and Welsh, the (Southern) Irish work fewer hours, get sick more often and stay away longer from work when they are ill. Three times as many men and twice as many women are in mental hospitals as their English counterparts, and they stay there longer. In the Irish Republic hospital admission rates are six times as high as in Britain for schizophrenia in young men, and ten times as high for alcoholism in all males.

The Irish Medicosocial Research Board considers that

much mental ill-health is associated with the peculiarities of Irish society: celibacy, late marriage, emigration of the young, and insufficient opportunities for rewarding work. Mental health is also affected by loneliness and the small holdings in the West of Ireland which are not only uneconomic but also isolate the often un-married and old men and women who live there.

The board cites as further evidence of mental ill-health in the Irish Republic that almost £1 in every £5 is spent on alcohol and tobacco, and the relative expenditure on drink is higher than in any other country in the world. The number of illnesses in the insured population has risen by 15 per cent in a six-year period, and the total number of days lost from work by 20 per cent. These sicknesses suggest that the main problems of life have been avoided rather than faced.

On the other hand, on average men live longer in the Republic than in England and Wales, though the reverse is true for women. Moreover, though alcoholism is common, the death rate from cirrhosis of the liver is surprisingly low.

ILLEGITIMACY

Illegitimacy is another important feature related to social class which has a profound influence on the individual's life. Most illegitimate children tend to be the firstborn of young mothers; generally, they weigh less at birth than legitimate children and their perinatal mortality rate is half as high again. Later on they tend to be backward in ability and achievement at school and to be rated by their teachers as unsettled or maladjusted. Nevertheless, the birth of an ille-gitimate child is often merely one sign of persistent social failure; among other things the parents tend to live in poor, overcrowded housing and have to move frequently.

The importance of the quality of rearing is shown by the progress of a group of illegitimate children included in the National Child Development Study. Most showed a depressing pattern in their subsequent development and the only exception was found among the 23 per cent of children who were adopted: not only did they thrive, but they tended to do better at school than legitimate children in normal families. Children brought up in slums or poor rural houses are known to be at a considerable disadvantage. Poor nutrition in the mother during pregnancy and in the child after birth probably leads to intellectual impairment, and an inadequate amount of play with and talking to adults leads to educational underachievement, particularly with speech and reading. Subsequently, backwardness in reading tends to be associated with antisocial behaviour and conduct problems, probably because the child is discouraged and loses his self-esteem, and antagonism (as shown by delinquency, vandalism and criminality) is the only means of compensation. Some schools produce many more delinquents than others – a feature related to the schools and not to the neighbourhood – but three quarters of all delinquent boys come from disrupted families.

SEPARATION

Disruption of the family, or a 'broken home', is a strong factor in producing antisocial behaviour, probably because of a loss or absence of the important bonds children form with one or both parents, or other adults. Much of the research into this subject has been done on children separated from their parents by admission to hospital or institutions, by pioneers such as Dr John Bowlby and Dr Michael Rutter. At first many separated children go through a phase of acute distress and crying, and this is succeeded by misery and apathy and, later, detachment and retarded development. A similar reaction is shown by children at the time that their parents get divorced. The effects of separation are most appreciable between the ages of six months and four years, and two groups appear to be particularly vulnerable: children who relate poorly to adults and other children, and boys compared with girls. The longer the separation, the greater the distress; but the effects can subsequently be reversed depending on the length and severity of the separation.

The key factor in the effects of separation is the stability of the family: children with the most favourable home environments are least affected by deprivation; those who are transiently separated from their parents during early life show an increased risk of later psychological disturbance only if there is associated family discord or stress; those in happy homes where one of the parents dies show only a very slight rise in later delinquency, which may reflect the grief in the surviving parent or the changed economic circumstance or both. On the other hand, some sort of bond between the child and both parents is probably necessary for normal psychological development.

There is no evidence that children of working mothers are particularly likely to become delinquent or psychiatrically disturbed. In fact, it has been said that such children may be less likely to develop these traits because the mothers' working reflects a high standard of family responsibility and care. Some types of happy separation of the child from its mother may prevent it from being affected by subsequent stressful separation, and, provided that a kind mother substitute is available, there is no evidence that the child comes to any harm. Moreover, in the average home the quality and quantity of maternal care are far better than in the average institution. Conversely, in the most loveless homes children may be so deprived that they fail to grow properly (probably due to undernutrition rather than to psychological causes, as was once thought) and here institutional care is the better alternative and is less likely to result in subsequent deviant behaviour.

QUALITY OF MOTHERING

The factor that stands out in research studies is the importance of the quality of mothering for the child's future. In immigrants to Britain in particular the absence of the 'extended family' whereby the mother can go to work leaving her children to be reared by the grandmother may be affecting the children's health. Research at St Mary's Hospital, Paddington, has shown that not only are the children of West Indian immigrants ill more often but that their development is usually well behind that of the children of their English neighbours living in the same deprived community. These children showed no evidence of physical injury or deformity and surprisingly, also, the immigrants were found to make as much, or more, use of the health services as their neighbours. But compared with English children, even those living in Paddington, many more of the immigrants had suffered from respiratory disorders or other minor illnesses, and they had also been admitted to hospital more often.

In a follow-up study of these immigrant babies when they were toddlers this pattern was still present. No fewer than a fifth of the three-year-old children had chest infections – a much higher incidence than in British children. But the medical team found the psychological picture even more disturbing. Not only was the West Indian children's verbal development poor, but they also failed to do well in simple manual dexterity tests. The psychologist generally had the impression of a conforming culture with emphasis on manners, cleanliness and obedience.

The reasons for these differences, the team thought, were disturbed environmental, cultural and family patterns. Overcrowding was the rule and there was little evidence of any contact with the community, while church attendance had declined. Over half the mothers were working, usually out of economic necessity since their husband's average wage was very low. The traditional baby-minders, the grandmothers, had mostly stayed behind in the West Indies. Parents were surprised and resentful that they had to pay for baby-minding at all, choosing people to do this on the grounds of cheapness and nearness to the home. On top of this, most mothers had at least one child living in the West Indies, while many were also pregnant at the time of the survey.

BATTERING

The statement made by Bowlby that 'mother love in infancy and childhood is as important for mental health as are vitamins and proteins for physical health' may have had the unintentional result of making social workers and others overkeen for children to be brought up in parental homes, however unsatisfactory these were. Thus quite recently many official agencies were returning 'battered' children to their natural parents, though 60 per cent of them are at risk of being injured again. Battering, now called 'non-accidental injury', is the fifth commonest cause of death between birth and the age of four years, the others being birth injuries, infections, congenital abnormalities and accidents, in that order (p. 291). Only recently has it been appreciated how commonly children are severely injured by their parents. In Britain this affects at least 4,000–5,000 children every year, of whom between 10 and 17 per cent die of their injuries and 30 per cent are permanently handicapped by brain damage. Even in the survivors emotional maladjustment may lead to slowed intellectual development. Put another way, non-accidental injury accounts for 10 per cent of children under the age of two years seen in a hospital casualty department and for 25 per cent of all fractures in children; serious burns and scalds are another frequent feature, while recently it has been shown that some children may be deliberately given large doses of powerful medicines.

Research in this field owes much to Dr Selwyn Smith and his team at Birmingham University, and has shown what makes a child liable to non-accidental injury. Typically the parents are young, in the lower social classes, have poor living conditions and work records, and live in marital disharmony. Between a third and two thirds of the parents were themselves battered as children; three quarters of the mothers conceive before marriage, and their average age at the birth of their first child is 19·7, compared with the national figure of 23·3. Most of the parents have an abnormal personality – 78 per cent and 64 per cent of the mothers and fathers, respectively – and half of the fathers are psychopaths. Eleven per cent of the mothers and 29 per cent of the fathers have criminal records.

The children subjected to this abuse tend to be the first- or second-born, in small families, and often they are not living with both natural parents. Half the children are under eighteen months old when they are injured.

INDIVIDUAL CHARACTERISTICS

Two of the most important characteristics in an individual's make-up seem to be the way in which his internal rhythms (or 'body clock') are set, and his personality, together with the way he responds to stress. About half of the population feel that there is a definite daily rhythm in their lives; some feel best soon after waking ('larks'), while others are at a peak later in the day ('owls'). Tests have shown that the inherent body rhythms differ between larks and owls: in the former, who tend to be introverts, the peak levels of body temperature and cortisol (an important hormone produced by the adrenal gland) occur earlier than in the owls, who tend to be extroverts.

From about 6.00 a.m. the body temperature rises more rapidly in larks than in owls, and the two levels are not the same until 2.00 p.m. Conversely from 6.00 p.m. the body temperature starts to fall in larks much more rapidly than in owls. Since the higher the body temperature the more efficient a normal person is, not surprisingly psychological tests prove that at 10.00 a.m. larks are more efficient than owls and less efficient at 3.00 p.m. German research has also shown that there is a strong social difference between the two types. Three quarters of labourers are larks, but only a quarter of white-collar workers.

These are just a few examples of how everybody's life is governed by built-in bodily rhythms. When uninfluenced by medical treatment, the commonest time of birth and death is around 3 a.m., the least frequent at tea-time; intellectually most people's peak is around midday, and women are at their most fertile on only one or two days every month. There are also many hidden rhythms: the body's ability to get rid of alcohol is maximal in the middle of the day; our teeth are looser during the night than they are in the day-time; and division of the cells making up the body reaches a peak between 1 and 3 o'clock in the morning. Because many rhythms follow a roughly twenty-four-hour pattern they are called 'circadian' – that is, they occur every day. But somebody deprived of reference points such as light and dark and the daily round tends to underestimate just how much time has passed, and follow a twenty-five-hour day.

Newborn babies do not have circadian rhythms but acquire them gradually as their brains mature; they are fully established by the second year of life. It is the upset of these rhythms produced by changing time-zones which produces the feeling of disorientation in somebody who has flown across the Atlantic (see p. 135). Iron-curtain politicians and some business firms now insist on at least a twenty-four-hour delay in important negotiations if those taking part have flown through some time-zones. Probably just as important is that men engaged in complex intellectual or physical tasks should perform these when they are at their peak; it is not too fanciful to foresee firms selecting owls for skilled procedures which have to be done in the late afternoon and larks for those in the early morning.

PSYCHOSOMATIC ILLNESS

Physicians in ancient Greece were aware that both the mind and the body are concerned in various illnesses. But about thirty years or so ago the concept of 'psychosomatic diseases' became fashionable, with the implication that psychological upsets *caused* some illnesses – in particular, peptic ulcer, migraine, ulcerative colitis and asthma. Doctors disagreed about this theory: for instance, some argued that ulcerative colitis (a prolonged illness with progressive damage to the lining of the intestine) could cause psychological changes rather than vice versa, while psychological tests by a research team in California showed that at the start of the illness there was no difference from normal in personality and mental stability of a group of patients who subsequently developed a converse behaviour pattern (no sense of urgency, no excessive competitive drive and no aggression).

Many experts do not accept this simple relation between personality and heart disease, although they believe that stress may be linked with the condition. Any theory that relates the increased prevalence of certain illnesses to the stress of modern life begs two questions: have the illnesses in fact become commoner (or are we just better at recognizing them?) and has stress really increased? 'The life of a physician in Birmingham is surely much less stressful than that of a peasant in the Yangtse Valley, with the ever-present menace of flood, famine, pestilence and war; or of the tribesman in equatorial Africa tortured by the taboo and sanction of primitive belief,' as Professor Sir Melville Arnott, a distinguished British cardiologist, once remarked.

The second of these questions is the easier to answer and, again, much of the research has been done on coronary disease, using a battery of psychological tests developed by a US naval psychiatrist, Lieutenant-Commander Richard Rahe, of San Diego in California. Each person completes a schedule which asks him a series of about sixty questions on recent changes in his life situation. These range from queries about his occupation, family life and marriage to questions about his earnings, personal habits and health. The answers are used to calculate a stress index for the individual. In a group of patients with coronary heart disease Rahe found that all had had the same stress index as the rest of the population – between 20 and 30 units – three years before the attack. But in the two years before the coronary the index rose, gradually at first but very steeply in the last six months. What was more, the final level of the index was proportional to the severity of the attack. Patients who died had an average index of almost 90, while for those who survived it was between 50 and 60. In every case the index rose well before the patient had any symptoms of coronary disease. After the attack the index gradually fell again until it was in the normal range a year later.

The medical team identified four particular life changes often occurring in the last six months: trouble with the boss, family upsets, minor law-breaking (such as parking tickets), and changes in working hours or conditions. Compared with the healthy group the coronary patients had had less personal success in this time, and had taken on fewer financial commitments, perhaps reflecting a basic insecurity.

Factors which cause severe stress in one country may have comparatively little effect in another. In North America, for example, the four most stressful changes in a person's life are death of a spouse, divorce, marriage and separation. In Mexico, on the other hand, the most stressful events are marriage, marital separation, deterioration in health and taking out a mortgage of over £4,000.

Rahe's findings have confirmed previous impressions that coronary patients are devoted to their work, tend to take too little leisure and are dissatisfied with their personal life. Low values in the stress index seemed to be related to holidays, which removed several of the important stresses in the Swedish patient's life situations. This may account for the success of medical 'reconditioning' centres in the Soviet Union and other communist countries. These centres are situated in quiet rural areas, and besides tackling any immediate stress aim to change the patient's whole attitude towards tension. Tried in Western Germany, such a centre was associated with 70 per cent reduction in absenteeism in the next two years.

STRESS

Further research into how stress may produce coronary disease has been carried out at the Middlesex Hospital by Dr Peter Taggart and a team who studied the stress of driving a car in ordinary traffic conditions and in racing. They found that stress releases large quantities of the adrenal hormone, noradrenaline, into the bloodstream, and this is accompanied by raised levels of fatty acids. The latter increase the stickiness of blood platelets and may also be converted into triglycerides, both of which predispose to atheroma formation (p. 44). During this stress even people with apparently normal hearts may show potentially dangerous alterations in heart rhythm. Similar changes accompanied milder stimuli such as lecturing or watching films.

Nevertheless, the theory that stress causes coronary disease is far from proved, and, even if it is a cause, heart disease is unlikely to be the sole way in which the body reacts to it. Research into other diseases which might reasonably be thought to be related to stress – such as migraine, ulcerative colitis and peptic ulcer – has yielded far from clear-cut cause-and-effect relationships. If anything, the converse has been found to be true: that these illnesses may *cause* the stress, rather than vice versa. Another approach has been to discover the effect of various types of undoubted stress on a group of people. Perhaps one of the mildest of these is living in high-rise flats. British service families living in flats in Germany were found to consult their doctors more often for psychoneurotic and respiratory disease than their counterparts living in houses, while menstrual irregularity was also commoner in women living in flats. More severe stresses may be temporary – as with riots, floods or air-raids – or long-lasting, as in the concentration camps.

At its most severe, short-term stress may kill. A frequent finding in coronary heart disease associated with sudden death is that in about half the instances this is linked with preceding social and psychological events. A common story is that the patient (who often has already had a coronary or a history of angina) has been depressed for several months before his final attack and is then exposed to 'acute arousal' – a sudden increase of work or activity, or anxiety and anger. The most common of these factors seems to be the departure of a child from the home or disappointment of parental expectations.

'Heart-break death'

A similar train of events seems to occur in the well-known 'heart-break death' that occurs in bereaved people. In the first six months after the death of a spouse the death rate is higher than otherwise expected – by 40 per cent for widowers, who are more likely to die unexpectedly than widows. The close relationships of many marriages are shown by the frequent occurrence of hallucinations of the dead spouse, which many people will admit to. These are commoner in people over forty, in professional people compared with others, and in those with a long and happy marriage. Nearly 5 per cent of widowers aged over forty-five die within six months of the death of their wife, mainly from coronary and other types of heart disease. Close relatives are also more likely to die after bereavement than similar people in the general population, while people who die after a bereavement tend to be younger than the relatives who predeceased them and younger than the usual age of death for the community in which they live. Conversely, elderly people often manage to stay alive until their birthdays, especially the notable anniversaries such as the ninetieth or hundredth. Deaths are significantly more frequent in the month after the birthday than in that before it.

Disasters – such as war, riots and floods – probably have a similar role in bringing out symptoms of existing illnesses or in hastening or precipitating sudden death from them. During the bombings in the Second World War doctors found that, though acute anxiety reactions were rare, deaths from peptic ulcer and coronary heart disease definitely increased. More recent evidence has come from a careful study of general practitioners' and hospital records of a group of people who were affected by the severe floods in Bristol in 1968, when five inches of rain fell on 10–11 July and about 3,000 properties were flooded. Research showed that in the succeeding year surgery attendances among those who had been flooded rose by 53 per cent, compared with a non-flooded group, and that hospital referrals more than doubled, though there was nothing to suggest any direct consequences of the flooding. The death rate in the flooded group rose by half, predominantly in people over sixty-five. All these changes were statistically significant for men, but not for women, and Dr Glin Benett, who carried out this research, asks whether men express their distress more in terms of physical ailments and women more in terms of emotional symptoms.

Concentration camps

Such research as has been done suggests that the effect of stress in increasing illness and death rates is relatively short-lived, probably lasting no longer than a year. But the possibility of longer-term effects has to be remembered, though whether these are due merely to stress or to hidden persisting physical damage is not yet known. A good example of this dilemma is provided by the experience of people surviving the German concentration camps. In Norway during the Second World War the Nazis imprisoned over 25,000 Norwegians for political reasons. Many prisoners endured the kind of brutal torture, starvation and mental stress that made these camps notorious.

At first after their release most prisoners seemed to recover rapidly. But ten years after the end of the war some ex-prisoners seemed to have relapsed or to have developed indefinite illnesses. There were also reports of broken marriages and of difficulties at work. Many ex-prisoners seemed to have withdrawn from human contact, and felt that they were misunderstood by doctors and psychiatrists. A full psychological and physical check-up at the University Hospital in Oslo was done on 227 people, including thirteen women, over half of whom had been subjected to systematic torture – very severe in many cases. The length of imprisonment had varied, but had averaged two and a half years.

The team found that though originally almost all of the prisoners had had stable personalities, this was no longer true: almost a fifth of them had become divorced and a similar proportion were unhappily married. Whereas within a year of their release most of them had been able to go back to work, at the time of the survey by Professor Axel Strøm a quarter of them were not employed at all. Two thirds had found it impossible to keep up with their jobs and had had to move to less demanding ones.

At the medical check-up a striking feature was that most of the ex-prisoners looked prematurely old. Many had some illness, the commonest being those affecting digestion, the heart or the lungs. One hundred and eighty had intellectual deterioration – loss of memory, lack of concentration, fatigue and mental disturbance. Tests showed that this was not a neurotic reaction to their appalling experiences, as might have been thought, but was due to a reduction in the size of the brain, proved by special X-rays and brain-wave recordings. Research in Japanese camps had shown that starvation causes the brain to swell, and it is thought that on return to normal conditions the brain then actually shrinks to less than its original size. Thus, though severe prolonged stress may have hidden effects after it has ended, this seems to be due to hidden physical effects at the time of the stress rather than to psychological ones.

Stress in women

Of the naturally recurring stresses the beginning of the menstrual period is recognized to be an important one (the premenstrual syndrome). Mental ability is reduced at this time, and normal behaviour altered, while a high proportion of women who attempt suicide do so then, and they are also much more liable to be involved in accidents. Moreover, in the mother's children, accidents and illness triggered off by a psychosomatic element such as asthma also increase just before and at the beginning of her menstrual period, probably as a reaction to the mother's mood.

These changes are temporary and seem to be related to the swings in the sex-hormone levels in the woman's bloodstream. Possibly similar, but much greater, swings are linked with puerperal depression, and certainly there is a high incidence of the premenstrual syndrome after such depression. Further confirmatory evidence of a relation to hormone levels is the characteristics of puerperal depressives during pregnancy: they tend to have an exceptionally favourable attitude towards motherhood (welcoming pregnancy, being free from any symptoms, and eager to breast-feed) with labile emotions throughout.

A breakdown in marriage is an obvious stress in women's lives, and, not surprisingly, two thirds of those whose marriages go on the rocks also have some breakdown in health. Almost all divorcees get some stress symptoms, usually described as 'nerves' or 'depression', but many women also develop more serious symptoms, such as severe loss of weight or sleeplessness, for which medical treatment is needed. Both types of symptom are worst at the time the marriage is breaking down and in the early separation period.

ROAD ACCIDENTS

Accidents of various kinds are a common cause of death for the various age groups (see p. 296). Road accidents, which cause a third of all deaths in men between the ages of fifteen and twenty-four, are a modern epidemic, causing over 250,000 deaths and 7·5 million injuries in the world in 1971. The figure for deaths in Britain for 1972 was no fewer than 7,762 deaths. A recent *Which* report has shown that in any year a man aged forty who drove vehicles had an increased risk of accidental death, as follows: motorbikes 90 per cent; scooters 20 per cent; and mopeds, bicycles and cars 10 per cent. Two fifths of the cyclists and moped riders and two thirds of the motorcyclists in the Consumer Association survey had had some sort of accident on their machines. In 1970 there were 2,300 riders of motorcycles and scooters fatally or seriously injured, and a further 1,000 people involved in these accidents, half of them pedestrians; for a boy who owns a motorcycle from sixteen to nineteen the risk of being killed or seriously hurt is 8 per cent.

Just under a half of fatal victims involving cars are pedestrians, often children or old people. To reduce these largely entails separating cars from pedestrians more – as by building more motorways, and pavements for rural roads – and designing vehicles which will cause fewer injuries. To reduce the fatalities in drivers means considering primary safety and safety factors in the car – defined respectively as design features which help prevent accidents from happening (such as good visibility and brakes), and those which minimize injury to the occupants (such as seat-belts). Some forty per cent of the deaths in car occupants are due to injury by gross deformation or penetration of the passenger compartment: 55 per cent of the occupants who die do so in head-on crashes, and the remainder in side, rear or rollover ones. The secondary safety factors which will help prevent these include seat-belts, collapsible steering columns, head rests, crushable front and back body sections, and reinforcing steel bars in the sides of the car.

Of all these factors, seat-belts are undoubtedly the most easily available means of cutting down deaths and serious injuries. Not only do they restrain the person in his seat and prevent his coming into contact with dangerous parts of the car, such as a shattered windscreen, but they prevent his being ejected outside it. Making the use of seat-belts compulsory in Australia cut down the death rate by 25 per cent, a figure corroborated by research on voluntary wearing of belts in Sweden. While the use of seat-belts remained voluntary in Britain only about 30 per cent of people wore seat-belts on motorways, 23 per cent on A-roads and 6 per cent in London, despite publicity campaigns. The new regulations making their use compulsory should do more to reduce the number of deaths and seriously injured than anything else since the drink-driving laws (see p. 219).

LONGEVITY

Excessive longevity is one of the perennial folk-legends that doctors are constantly having to destroy for the sake of truth. Stories of so many thousands of centenarians living in this or that country always have two things in common; the country is remote and its inhabitants largely illiterate. They may also be fond of classifying everything in decades – 80–90, 90–100, 100–110, with the figures usually rounded up. In fact, according to the *Guinness Book of Records*, the oldest fully authenticated person ever was Pierre Jonbert, who lived 113 years 124 days (from 1701 to 1814), while the 1971 census records 2,450 people in Britain over the age of 100.

Apart from national pride, there are several reasons why legends of immense longevity have grown up. Some people take their father's Christian names; they may falsify their ages to avoid call-up; and mental changes in old age may lead them to mistake their true ages. Add to this the fact that in some countries there is no distinct difference between the seasons and the difficulty of keeping accurate records is obvious. Even in the advanced countries reliable birth and death certificates have been a feature only of the last hundred years; using them, together with proof of name change in women, it has been possible to dispute many extravagant claims about longevity.

Despite all these reservations, however, there do seem to be verified areas where centenarians are unexceptional, notably in the valley of Vilcabamba in Ecuador, where out of a population of 819 there are nine people over 100 years (three of them said to be over 120). Such factors as have been identified are a low-calorie, vegetarian diet, vigorous physical activity, tranquillity and an equable climate, but other features include consumption of up to sixty cigarettes and two cupfuls of neat rum a day.

In the developed countries there is a definite tendency for the offspring of long-lived parents to survive longest – particularly for the sons of long-lived mothers. The main reason for longevity seems to be a diminished rate of decay in middle age rather than excessive prolongation of the range of life.

SUICIDE

The commonest feature among people who commit suicide is the history of a broken home. Most suicides have vulnerable and abnormal personalities, but only a third have obvious mental illness – depression carrying the highest risk. Despite world-wide study of why people kill themselves, done increasingly by specialized units, we still have little idea why some do it and others do not, and what remains is a mass of statistics.

All over the world something like 1,000 people commit suicide every day. Numerically it is commonest in the over-fifty-fives, but the highest proportion of deaths from suicide occur in twenty-five to thirty-four-year-olds, with a peak frequency in the early summer. In order of frequency the countries where suicide is commonest are Hungary, Finland, Austria and Czechoslovakia. The only two countries in which the rates are falling are Japan and Britain, possibly because in the former recent cultural changes have laid less stress on dishonour and its expiation while in the latter the ready and wide availability of the Samaritan centres has been claimed as an important factor. The stereotype of Sweden as the country with the highest rate has been untrue for many years but may have arisen from the absence of prejudice against suicide there and ready availability of scrupulously accurate figures, in Britain, for example, possibly only half of all true suicides are reported as such. Nevertheless, these figures almost certainly do reflect some kind of real national differences, as suggested by the finding that the suicide rates among immigrants to the USA still reflect the rate of their country of origin.

Compared with the lower social classes those in the upper ones are more likely to kill themselves, and doctors in particular are two and a half times as likely to kill themselves as all men and one and a half times as likely as their social equals. In Britain 6 per cent of all doctors who die before sixty-five kill themselves, and the suggestion is that the availability of poisonous drugs, the increased incidence of addiction to alcohol or dangerous drugs, or both, and the regular acquaintance with death all contribute to this. American research has shown that the doctor-suicide tends to be a compulsively competitive and ambitious man who usually works in a peripheral branch of medicine, often with chronically ill patients who rarely make a good recovery.

PARASUICIDE

All these facts comprise the 'classical' associations of suicide. But recent research has focused particularly on attempted suicide; even successful suicide may not have been intentional and sometimes there is no clear distinction between life-events in the successful and the non-successful suicide. The latter is now often called parasuicide, or 'self-poisoning', to indicate that the person has taken too much of a poisonous substance believing only that it will be noxious. The term self-poisoning also indicates that medicines (sleeping pills, tranquillizers and pain-killers) have now replaced the older methods of violence and coal gas.

Few laymen probably realize the extent to which most countries are faced with an epidemic of self-poisoning: every year some 100,000 adults are treated in hospitals in England and Wales for this condition, which is responsible for 15 per cent of all acute medical admissions. In some units between 1960 and 1971 the total of cases increased by 350 per cent and is continuing to rise at the rate of 15 per cent a year. All this means that the ratio of parasuicide to completed suicide, which was 10:1 in the 1960s, had risen to 36:1 in the early 1970s.

We owe much of our knowledge of parasuicide to Professor Neil Kessel, now of Manchester University, whose research was carried out in the special Poisons Treatment Centre at Edinburgh. He found that the peak age group for parasuicide was twenty to twenty-five, and, whereas the rate for men remained fairly constant between twenty and sixty-four, that in women dropped steeply after they were twenty-five. Less than half his patients had really wanted to die at the time of their attempt, and in only a fifth of all cases had the attempt been really determined. The central factor in most histories was disorganization – a disorganized life pattern, a disorganized marriage and living in a disorganized district. Alcoholism was often associated – heavy drinking occurring in 70 per cent of cases – while a quarter of the men and a fifth of the women had no psychiatric illness. A history of a broken home was common, with one of the parents having been abnormally absent owing to separation, hospital admission or death. The motives for parasuicide included troubled relationships with other people, distress arising from within, material problems – such as money and housing – and 'no reason' or 'don't know'.

Finally other research has shown that people who attempt suicide on impulse are more likely to repeat the attempt than those where the episode was planned, as are people with personality disorders compared with those without them.

There is also a role for imitation. For example, carbon copies of the suicides of the poet Chatterton and Goethe's character Werther have been common. A recent illustration of the phenomenon was provided by a 268-day news blackout in Detroit: during this period, the suicide rate was the lowest for five years, being 20 per cent below the mean figure when newspapers were being published. The fact that parasuicide so often represents a 'cry for help' was shown at the time of the hospital doctors' industrial action in 1975–76, when the number of cases was reported to have fallen dramatically. Presumably the (mistaken) idea that they would not have been treated led potential parasuicides to think again.

Chapter 2

DIET AND DISEASE

MOST of us enjoy food, and even those who get no pleasure from it have to choose every day whether and what to eat and how much. The close connection between food and health has always been recognized in folklore and still is in advertising and popular journalism – 'tell me what you eat: I will tell you what you are', said Brillat-Savarin.* The public seems to have a never-ending interest in new diets guaranteed to preserve or restore youthful vitality and in new scare stories about the dangers of food additives, cooking processes or farming methods. Large-scale medical research into the relation between diet and disease is comparatively new, but some facts are now undisputed and many myths and fads have been demolished.

Dietary habits are difficult to change, and it is futile to expect people to eat unpalatable food unless they are convinced that the change is essential. Only too often medical research findings – certainties, probabilities and long shots – are not put into the perspective of their implications for the expectation of life and its enjoyment.

The most dramatic effect of food is that occasionally it may be a cause of sudden death by choking, usually on a large piece of meat. The typical victim is middle-aged or elderly, wears dentures, and has been drinking heavily. While trying to swallow some solid food he suddenly collapses in complete silence: death is often falsely ascribed to a heart attack. Some 700 to 1,000 deaths from this cause are thought to occur each year in the USA but the number occurring in Britain is not known.

* *Philosopher in the Kitchen*, Penguin, 1970.

OBESITY

Even small variations from the theoretical ideal diet can have striking effects if they are maintained for years; and this is nowhere more apparent than in the most obvious and most common result of a faulty diet, obesity or overweight. Only tooth decay matches the frequency of obesity among the physical disorders affecting people living in developed countries today. Obesity is also potentially the most serious western disease: any degree of overweight may shorten life and is associated with a higher risk of unpleasant illnesses from arthritis to heart disease. There is little scientific support for the common belief that fat people often eat less than average; it is certainly true that everyone can lose weight if they eat less.

So to put it simply obesity is directly linked with the amount of food eaten – and its type, for starchy and sugary foods are specially likely to lead to gains in weight. Large quantities of fat are nauseating (except when the body needs unusually large amounts of energy, as in polar exploration) while pure protein actually needs more energy to metabolize it than it provides, which is why it forms the basis of most slimming diets. Few comparative statistics have been kept of the prevalence of obesity over the years, but it seems to be associated with affluence. Prints from Dr Johnson's days show rich people corpulent in their twenties and thirties, contrasting with their skinny retainers and servants in the background. In our own day it is a commonplace that the general population in countries with the highest levels of material prosperity, such as Western Germany and the USA, tend to be more obese than those in countries which have been less successful economically.

Unfortunately there is little likelihood that any very fat person will stay slim even if he or she does succeed in losing a lot of weight, despite the efforts of doctors to scare their patients with phrases such as 'you're digging your grave with your teeth', frequent books and magazine articles devoted to slimming, and the promotion of commercial slimming foods. Most people can lose weight for a few weeks; but less than a quarter can permanently reverse a lifetime pattern of eating and stay slim.

It is not necessarily easy for people to decide whether or not they are overweight. Formal medical definitions – a body-fat content exceeding 20 per cent in men and 30 per cent in women – may be fine for scientists but are of little help to the woman worried about her contours. The layman might think that obesity could be measured merely by weighing oneself, but again the problem cannot be solved that simply. Weighing ignores the size of the body frame and the other two heavy components of the body, bone and muscle. Inevitably, weight tables are based on averages, often taken from a particular group, such as Army recruits or people taking out a life insurance policy; also they often ignore the fact that the average weight for height gradually increases over the years.

As a rule of thumb, doctors still use height/weight tables adjusted for sex and for small, medium and large body frames; these make no allowance for any increase in weight with age, since theoretically the ideal weight is reached by the age of twenty and should not increase after this. For greater accuracy, callipers can be used to measure the thickness of the fold of skin just above the back of the elbow.

Obesity needing treatment is present in anybody who is 10 per cent or more over his ideal weight. On this definition, it affects between 2 and 5 per cent of children, at least 20 per cent of young men and women, and over 50 per cent of people over the age of forty. Surveys in London general practices have shown that overall 56 per cent of the women and 52 per cent of the men were at least 15 per cent above their ideal weight; no fewer than 25 per cent and 18 per cent of them were, respectively, at least 30 per cent overweight.

Although experts still disagree, probably obesity is commoner in women than in men, and in working people compared with professional ones. Smokers tend to be lighter than non-smokers, though on average both groups are over-weight – in one survey, by 15 and 28 lb. respectively (p 256). Surprisingly, people who smoke heavily – over thirty-five cigarettes a day – are more obese than moderate smokers. This may be because heavy smoking is linked with heavy drinking or excessive consumption of sugary tea. In smokers the usual rise in weight during adult life tends to stop by the age of thirty-seven, whereas in non-smokers this continues until fifty.

The basic cause of obesity is quite simple: at some time the body has taken in more calories than it could put out. This principle of an imbalance between input and output applies even to those excessively rare cases where 'gland troubles' – that is, endocrine disorders – are also present. Certainly obesity may often occur in people with, for example, under-activity of the thyroid gland (myxoedema) but it still means that the patient has eaten too much for his or her needs, which characteristically are lower than normal in this disease. And it is important to emphasize that in the vast majority of people with obesity no associated disorder is present whatsoever.

This idea of an imbalance is useful in differentiating be-tween the usual cause of obesity in childhood and that in adult life. Stated simply, fat children usually overeat; fat adults usually take too little exercise and go on eating the same amount of food. Furthermore, a layer of fat acts like lagging and prevents loss of body-heat in cold weather and so further reduces food requirements. Obese people are not necessarily gluttons: surprisingly little excess food may lead to obesity. Only 100 calories above requirements every day (two slices of bread, a medium-sized boiled potato or a large apple) may result in a weight gain of 10 lb. a year.

Recent research has shown that up to the age of one year the number of fat cells in the body can probably increase, but thereafter this remains constant for the rest of one's life. So doctors can now classify obesity into two types, though the relative frequency of each is still not known. In the first type the total number of fat cells in the body is increased; in the second the individual fat cells are larger than normal. All obese people have larger individual fat cells in their bodies; but there is now good evidence that those who gained weight excessively during the first year of life also have more fat cells than normal. Fat babies tend to become fat children. The more quickly a child gained weight in infancy, the more likely he is to be overweight in later childhood – a much better guide in fact than the weight of his parents. Even more seriously, 80 per cent of childhood obesity persists into adult life.

Research into risks associated with obesity in early childhood has started only recently. But it is already known to be associated with an increased risk of respiratory infections serious enough to last for a minimum of three days and needing a doctor's attention. 'Cot deaths' may also be commoner in fat infants than in ones of normal weight. In later childhood, obesity may produce obvious mechanical effects such as knock knees and flat feet, while in rare and very severe cases it may reduce breathing sufficiently to produce serious and persistent sleepiness – the so-called 'Pickwickian syndrome', named after Dickens's fat boy.

The risks of obesity in adult life have been studied much more fully. Overall, the mortality of men 10 per cent or more overweight is one fifth higher than average; the corresponding increases for people 20 per cent and 30 per cent overweight are about one third and two fifths. In women the risks are slightly less: 9, 20 and 30 per cent, respectively. These increased risks are associated particularly with deaths from diabetes (130 per cent excess mortality in men) and from vascular disease (30 per cent excess for coronary disease and 50 per cent excess for vascular disease of the central nervous system in men). Other, smaller, increases in risk are found for pneumonia, diseases of the digestive system, and accidents and homicide.

But obesity is also linked with an increased incidence of troublesome illnesses that do not necessarily shorten life.

The first type of these complications are those associated with the sheer mechanical problems of excess weight, including osteoarthritis, wear and tear changes affecting the weight-bearing joints in the legs (particularly the hips and knees), flat feet, and varicose veins in the legs.

Two types of hernia are also commoner in obese people: the so-called 'ventral' hernia and diaphragmatic hernia. In the first, the thick layer of fat on the front of the abdomen causes the muscles to become separated in the middle, allowing the intestines or other contents of the abdominal cavity to pass through in a pouch formed by lining tissue of the cavity (the peritoneum). In the second type, too much fat in the abdominal cavity raises the pressure there, so pushing out the stomach or other organs into the chest through one or more openings between it and the abdomen.

The second type of illness associated with obesity is due to its effects on metabolism – that is, the general workings of the body. Diabetes is four times commoner in obese than in lean adults. Excessively fat people have high blood levels of insulin, the hormone produced by the pancreas that regulates the level of sugar in the bloodstream. Probably the continual strain on the pancreas, which has to produce much higher quantities of insulin than normal, eventually exhausts the gland and so leads to diabetes. But obesity also interacts with other factors, environmental and genetic, in producing diabetes. Thus diabetes is three times as common in the brothers and sisters of people with the disease, but its highest incidence is found in the obese brothers and sisters of non-obese diabetics.

Obesity is also linked with raised levels of cholesterol and other fatty substances in the bloodstream. This may account for the increased incidence of gallstones in fat people, and also its link with atherosclerotic disease, which affects the blood-vessels (p. 44 and p. 299). This tendency, together with the fact that obesity is definitely related to raised blood pressure, could be expected to increase the risk of disease of the coronary arteries (p. 300). This proves to be the case, though the link is not between fatness and actual coronary thrombosis (a blood clot in the arteries) but with the development of angina pectoris (pain originating from the heart muscle) or with sudden death. In other words, obesity throws an extra strain on the heart.

All these results emphasize our continuing ignorance of why some people eat so much more than others, and so become obese. 'In general it can be said that eating is pleasant, it helps to pass the time, and can cost little. It also can be indulged in at will and does not interfere with the lives of others.' The truth of Dr John Anderson's apparently flippant remark has been reinforced by some recent research in New York. In this experiment, groups of lean and obese people were asked to take their meals as a kind of mush, or 'liquid formula', of which they could get as much as they liked from a machine. During the experiment the calorie content of the formula was changed, and each person's intake was measured, though nobody knew that either of these changes was being made. When the formula was changed, lean people adjusted the amount of diet to keep their weight constant; on the other hand, fat adults took in only a fraction of the calories they needed to keep their weight constant, and so invariably lost weight. This is unlike the situation in cigarette smoking, where if smokers are given low-nicotine cigarettes they adapt by taking longer puffs and smoking more.

This study also reinforced modern views that obesity in childhood may differ from that in adults: the two obese children included in the above study either kept their weight constant or actually increased it.

DENTAL DECAY

The second commonest physical disorder, dental decay (or caries), is far more frequent than most people realize. By the age of two half the children in Britain have bad teeth, and on average a child of four has at least four decayed teeth and thereafter acquires another one for every year of his child-hood. Hence dentures for children are no longer rare, while the average adult in England and Wales who still has his own teeth left has about seventeen teeth which are filled and two which need restoration, and one in every two adults has a tooth that needs extracting.

Dental decay is due to an attack on the enamel surface of the teeth by bacteria which grow in the stagnating food debris left between the teeth after a meal. These bacteria act on simple sugars in this debris to form acid, a process which may take only a few minutes. Normally the saliva in the mouth would neutralize this acid but it is prevented from doing so by dental plaque – a scum composed of bacteria and the tooth surface. The frequency of dental caries is related to how much refined carbohydrate the population eats; in the developing countries caries is relatively rare in the general population and much commoner in the rich individuals who eat a European-type diet. The chief culprits are cakes and sweets, which contain the simpler sugars. How often these are eaten is more important than how much; eating sweets between meals is particularly harmful, and toffees are a notorious culprit. Children who are taught at schools which sell sweets in tuckshops have more dental decay than those at schools which do not.

Another common cause of rampant caries in early child-hood is the hollow feeder dummy, which is often sweetened with undiluted rose-hip syrup, honey, golden syrup or sugar. Mothers often give their babies a bottle to suck to keep them quiet at night and the jet of sweetened liquid may rapidly cause gross decay of the milk teeth. Some vitamin supplements now carry warnings against giving them to infants in this way.

Apart from stopping snacks between meals, caries may be controlled in two other ways. Dental plaque can be removed by vigorous brushing, eating fresh fruit or vegetables, and rinsing the mouth round with water at the end of meals. The presence of very small quantities of fluoride in drinking water undoubtedly protects substantially against caries, not only in children but also in adults. In areas where fluoride is present naturally the incidence of caries is reduced by a half; people aged sixty-five in Hartlepool, where the water naturally contains fluoride, had the same average dental decay as nineteen-year-olds in York, where the water does not. In the few areas in Britain where fluoride has been added artificially the degree of protection has been the same. A particularly convincing demonstration of the benefits of fluoridation was provided at Kilmarnock, where fluoridation was started in 1956 and ended in 1962. In children born during this period dental decay was reduced by half the normal figure, but in those born after it the caries rate again went up to the usual national level.

Despite much experience with artificial fluoridation in other countries no harm has been shown to result from the small quantities used. People can be protected against caries by the addition of one part per million, and protection does not increase with higher concentrations. At two parts per million mottling of the teeth can just be detected by an expert and at three parts per million this becomes obvious. Much higher concentrations may cause hardening of the bones and a hunchback deformity, the condition of 'fluorosis' seen in a few parts of India and the Middle East. Even so, concentrations of forty parts per million and above are needed to cause fluorosis, which has never been seen even in those Western countries with drinking water supplies naturally containing levels as high as six to eight parts per million.

The strong opposition to fluoridation of drinking water in Britain ignores the safety of low concentrations of fluoride and also that over forty million people in the USA have now been drinking artificially fluoridated water for some years without any harm. Moreover, of all the ways of giving this element, fluoridation is the easiest and the cheapest. Calculations in America showed that spending $100,000 on water fluoridation would prevent 660,000 cavities; on fluoride applied to the gums 60,000 cavities; on fluoride toothpaste 25,600 cavities; and on tooth-filling 16,606 cavities. Yet so far in Britain public opinion has refused to sanction this measure, an attitude which led Sir George Godber, then Chief Medical Officer of the Department of Health and Social Security, to comment: 'the baseless opposition to this humane and safe measure in Britain makes a mockery of one aspect of the care of children's health'. In 1976 an expert team from the Royal College of Physicians of London examined the pros and cons of fluoridation and recommended the addition of fluoride to water supplies where the concentration was less than one part per million. Advice to the opponents of fluoridation was also given by a leading article in the *British Medical Journal*.

In one African tribe an attack of dental caries is considered sufficient grounds for divorce. If one of the children has decayed teeth he is forbidden to feed from the family pot; he sits forlornly in the corner of the hut and dines alone. Under these rules almost all the marriages in Britain would be broken and all but a few children would eat alone . . .

THE 'DISEASES OF CIVILIZATION'

Obesity and tooth decay are not the only hazards of the modern diet, and anyone concerned about the effect of food on his health needs to pay attention to other things apart from sugar and the total calorie intake. As infectious diseases have been conquered by modern medicine, heart disease, stroke and cancer have become more important causes of death. Medical authorities still do not agree about how important the composition of the diet is in causing these 'diseases of civilization'. The three major theories which link disease with features of the modern diet incriminate animal fats, cane sugar and the low-fibre diet.

Cholesterol and animal fat

The best-known theory of the three is the animal fat/cholesterol explanation for coronary thrombosis. A vast amount of research has been done in the last twenty years into this disorder, which is now by far the most common form of death before the age of sixty in Western society. Each year fatal heart-attacks due to coronary thrombosis account for one in every four deaths in Britain, and not a few victims are men in their thirties and forties. Coronary thrombosis kills three times more people than die from road accidents, lung cancer and breast cancer added together: and in addition the arterial disease that leads to coronary thrombosis affects blood-vessels elsewhere in the body, causing strokes, high blood pressure and gangrene.

As long ago as the mid-nineteenth century the German pathologist Virchow showed that patches of yellow, mushy material could accumulate beneath the inner lining of arteries. These deposits, called atheroma from the Greek *athere* (mush), disturb the smooth blood flow in the arteries, and blood-clots – thrombi – form, narrowing the bore of the vessels. A heart-attack or stroke occurs when a thrombosis finally blocks the artery, cutting off the blood supply from the heart muscle or from part of the brain, respectively.

Virtually everyone in a Western society has some atheroma in their arteries, and the amount increases with age. Certain factors (p. 299) increase the individual risk of atheroma being severe enough to end in coronary thrombosis, including male sex, a family tendency to the disease, cigarette smoking, high blood pressure, diabetes and obesity. The debatable factor is the role of the diet. Atheroma consists largely of cholesterol, a complex crystalline alcohol that is one of the most common substances in the body. The amount of cholesterol in the blood serum varies widely in healthy people, but research has clearly shown that communities which are relatively free of atheroma and so of coronary thrombosis have low blood-cholesterol levels and usually eat diets low in cholesterol and animal fats. Conversely, communities with a high incidence of atheroma generally have high cholesterol levels and tend to eat high-cholesterol diets.

For any individual, the higher the level of cholesterol in the blood the more likely he is to have a coronary thrombosis. Most men in a Western society have serum cholesterol levels in the range 130 to 260 mg./100 ml.: the likelihood of coronary thrombosis has been shown to bear a 'linear relationship to the cube of the cholesterol value'; in other words, a man with a cholesterol level of 300 is five times more likely to have a coronary thrombosis than a man with otherwise equal risk factors (smoking, weight, etc.) whose cholesterol is only 180. Logically the key to prevention of coronary thrombosis would seem to lie in reducing the serum cholesterol level, by modifying the diet. In the late 1940s there was apparently every prospect of success from such an approach, but now we know that the problem has no easy solution.

The first difficulty is that lowering the serum cholesterol level is not simply a matter of reducing the amount of cholesterol in the diet. Four fifths of the cholesterol in the body is formed by the liver from other foodstuffs. Cholesterol itself is an essential constituent of the mitochondria within cells, the cell membranes themselves, and the sheaths around nerve fibres. One eighth of the dry weight of the brain is cholesterol. To reduce the serum cholesterol level demands changes in the overall composition of the diet and the total calorie intake.

The effect of diet on cholesterol is closely linked with the type of fat eaten and the chemical composition of fat in different parts of the body. There are two main forms of human fat. Many vital structures within cells, the bulk of all nerve tissues, and the brain itself are made of 'structural' fat. The second type is storage fat, which acts as an energy reserve and insulates against loss of heat: this is found in layers beneath the skin, around the kidneys, and in the breasts and buttocks. Chemically, the composition of the two forms of fat is quite distinct, the essential difference being the type of fatty acid they contain. Fatty acids are long chains of carbon atoms with an acidic group at one end. If the carbon chain has the maximum number of hydrogen atoms attached to it the acid is termed 'saturated'. If the full complement of hydrogen atoms is not present the acid is 'unsaturated', and if more than one pair of carbon atoms lacks these it is called 'polyunsaturated'. Structural fat consists of glycerol, phosphorus and unsaturated fatty acids. Storage fat, on the other hand, does contain some saturated fatty acids. Cholesterol is found associated with both forms of fat.

Storage fat is characteristic of animals, and almost all the saturated fat in the diet comes from animal products such as butter, milk and meat. Domestic animals contain much more saturated fat than wild animals, while vegetables usually contain unsaturated fat – the dietary sources being nuts, berries, seeds and vegetable oils. Cholesterol is found in milk and milk products, and eggs are particularly rich in it.

A diet in which most of the fat is polyunsaturated and the cholesterol level is low undoubtedly lowers the blood-cholesterol level. This is also, claim its proponents, the 'natural' diet of man, who in primitive societies relies much more on nuts, berries and seeds than on meat, which is rare. Even meat-eaters such as Eskimoes live on wild animals whose fat is much more unsaturated than that of domestic animals.

Essentially, then, the animal-fat theory of coronary artery disease has three steps. Coronary artery disease is found only in communities with high blood-cholesterol levels, and whose diets are rich in saturated animal fat and cholesterol. Communities with little or no coronary disease have low blood-cholesterol levels and live on a natural diet low in saturated fats and cholesterol and high in polyunsaturated fats. Such a diet, which lowers the cholesterol level, should reduce the incidence of coronary disease in the community.

This argument is intellectually attractive, and diets designed to cut the risk of coronary disease have been widely promoted, especially in the USA and Scandinavia, for over twenty years. The results have been disappointing.

The essential feature of an unsaturated fat diet is that milk, cream, eggs, butter, cheese, dripping, suet and many forms of meat are rationed and replaced by margarine, vegetable oils, some nuts and plant products. It soon became apparent that such diets would lower the level of cholesterol in the blood serum by about 10–15 per cent, but that any further reduction would require severe restriction of calories as well. Such 'nature' diets tend to be more popular among people who are health-conscious – and who tend to take plenty of exercise, to be non-smokers, and to be of average or below average weight. To test the effect of the diet scientifically the difference in diet should be the only variation between two large groups of people otherwise identical in the features known to affect the risk of coronary thrombosis. Medical research workers have found it difficult to assemble the volunteers necessary for such large-scale comparisons and to persuade them to follow the rules of the experiment for years at a time. The diet is unattractive and somewhat unpalatable, and many of the experiments have foundered because of 'cheating' by the participants. Only about half a dozen reasonably large trials have been continued long enough for the results to be valid, though several more are in progress. In general, the diets given in these trials have been effective in reducing the cholesterol level by about 15 per cent and over periods of up to twelve years the group on the diet have shown a reduction in coronary heart disease.

Perhaps the best-known experiment is one that did not fulfil the strict criteria of a scientific trial: the 'Anti-Coronary Club' in New York. Men were enrolled into the club if they seemed at risk of coronary disease because they were either overweight or had a high blood-cholesterol level. The controls were men of the same age seen at one of the city's cancer-detection centres and found not to be at special risk. The club members were put on to a low-cholesterol, low-saturated-fat diet; the controls were given no dietary advice. After nearly 4,000 man-years of experience, thirty-two heart attacks had occurred in the controls compared with only seventeen in the slightly larger group of club members.

Of the strict dietary trials, the best results have come from a Finnish study on several thousand patients in two large mental hospitals. Mortality from coronary thrombosis among men on the diet was only half that of the control group: but curiously in this and some other trials the overall death rates in the two groups were not significantly different, the men on the diet showing an increased mortality from non-cardiac disease. All trials have agreed that any beneficial effect of a low-cholesterol diet is much more definite in men than in women.

The major problem in organizing such long-term trials is to maintain the enthusiasm and interest of the participants for their unpalatable diet. Motivation is much stronger, however, among people who have recovered from a coronary thrombosis and wish to avoid a recurrence. There have been several trials of dietary reduction of cholesterol in such groups, but again the results have been somewhat equivocal. Whereas trials in the USA, Hungary and Oslo showed a reduction in further coronary episodes in the groups on the diet, three studies in London (including one by the Medical Research Council) failed to show a statistically significant benefit.

So after twenty years of experimentation and research there is still no uniformity of medical opinion. Clearly diet has some part in causing coronary artery disease and equally clearly altering the diet has some beneficial effect on the risk of heart-attacks; but how much emphasis should be laid on the dietary factor is still uncertain. In Britain the trend in recent years has been to abandon strict dietary regimens in favour of general advice on moderation in animal fats and milk products, while the research effort has swung to the investigation of drugs which lower the serum cholesterol level. Two such drugs, clofibrate and cholestyramine, have been under trial for some years but their use has proved disappointing in preventing further episodes of coronary disease in patients who have had one attack. Their place in preventing disease in healthy people is still being investigated.

Refined sugar

These disappointing results of attempts to prevent coronary artery disease by reducing the serum cholesterol led research workers to look for other features of the Western diet which might be responsible for the increased frequency of cardiovascular disease. The pioneer in this field was Professor John Yudkin, of London University, who in the late 1950s drew attention to the close correlation between the amount of refined sugar consumed by a community and its incidence of coronary heart disease. Sugar was unknown in Europe before the seventeenth century, but since then consumption has risen to the present-day level of about 1 kg. per person per week – nearly 10 per cent of the total calorie intake. Most of this rise has occurred in the twentieth century, paralleling the rise in heart disease. This suggestive epidemiological evidence has been supported by research studies showing that the proportion of sugar in the diet appreciably affects the amount and composition of fatty substances (lipids), particularly glycerides, in the blood. Could this alteration in the lipid pattern be responsible for the development of atheroma in the arterial walls?

Just as with the animal fat/cholesterol theory, however, careful research studies showed that there was no simple solution. The Medical Research Council asked a group of epidemiologists and heart specialists to examine the theory. Their report showed that there was no significant difference in the amounts of sugar taken by men with coronary thrombosis and those consumed by an otherwise comparable group with unrelated conditions such as hernia or bronchitis.

There were, however, more smokers among the patients with heart disease than the controls: and the MRC suggested that any slight tendency for them to consume a lot of sugar could probably be explained by the known tendency for heavy smokers to drink a lot of sweet tea.

There are excellent medical reasons for advising a low sugar intake: its role as a cause of tooth decay and its contribution to the excessive calorie intake of people who are overweight. But there seems no convincing evidence that sugar is an important factor in causing coronary heart disease.

High- and low-residue diets

The most recent medical attack on the Western diet, like its predecessors, is based on epidemiological evidence. Coronary heart disease is the main killing disease in advanced countries, but there are many other 'diseases of civilization' which are common in urban societies but are rare among rural peasants in underdeveloped countries: stomach ulcers, varicose veins, appendicitis and chronic constipation and its complications such as diverticular disease of the colon. Most of these diseases resemble coronary thrombosis in having become common only in the present century.

A group of British doctors with extensive practical experience in Africa first drew attention to the absence of these diseases among Africans living in tribal communities. Among the many thousands of such people seen at mission hospitals these diseases are seldom if ever seen. The African group suggested that there is one fundamental difference between the modern diet and that eaten by the rural African: the latter is the natural one for which man's digestive tract has been designed by evolution. Contrasted with the Western one, the African diet has a high residue of indigestible material, which is eliminated in the faeces.

Until the end of the nineteenth century even the privileged classes in Europe and the USA ate a lot of unprocessed food, the main sources of energy being wholemeal bread and other wheat products. Such a diet contains a substantial amount of indigestible vegetable fibres. About 1880 two changes began: roller milling removed most of the fibre from wheat, and for the first time bread became white; and cheap refined cane sugar began to make a significant contribution to most people's diet. Within twenty years white bread, sugar and potatoes had become the staple sources of energy. The effect of this change was to reduce the amount of vegetable fibre in the diet, so reducing the bulk of indigestible matter to be eliminated from the body.

Experts on the large bowel, notably a London surgeon, Mr Neil Painter, argue that now the average Western man has such a small mass of faeces passing through the colon that the bowel muscle cannot propel it along. As a result the faeces pass through the colon slowly and sluggishly, high pressures are generated by muscular spasm, and eventually the muscular wall of the colon is damaged. This damage leads to the formation of small pouches or diverticula in the colon wall. Certainly the time taken for the faeces to pass through the colon is much longer in people in advanced countries than in rural Africans, and diverticular disease is now an almost invariable finding in middle-aged and elderly people in Britain and the USA, and so are its symptoms of chronic constipation, attacks of lower abdominal pain and feelings of distension. Severe diverticular disease may cause internal bleeding and episodes of inflammation of the bowel. The condition can, says Painter, be relieved or reversed by the simple expedient of restoring to the diet the fibre in which it is deficient. Indeed, within the last two or three years his treatment of diverticular disease by giving the patients vegetable fibre as bran has been proved effective and been accepted by most gastro-enterologists.

What is much more arguable is the view advanced by some of this group that the Western fibre-deficient diet is the underlying cause of almost the whole range of the diseases of civilization. The distinguished surgeon, Mr Denis

Burkitt, argues, for example, that varicose veins and piles are caused by repeated episodes of raised abdominal pressure in people straining to overcome constipation due to the low-fibre diet. Equally plausible explanations have been devised to link the low-fibre diet with bowel cancer, peptic ulcer and appendicitis, while dietary fibre is also said to influence lipid metabolism and so to be relevant in the causation of coronary heart disease. Apart from the geographical distribution of these diseases, such theories are still only hypotheses and they have not yet received widespread medical support.

Frequency of meals

One more characteristic of modern eating habits needs to be considered: the frequency of meals. Again, the starting point for the discussion is the model of primitive man spending his day gathering and eating seeds, berries and fruit. Is man naturally a herbivorous animal, nibbling all day long, or a natural carnivore, gorging himself once every day or more?

All the evidence favours nibbling. In animals (including chickens, rabbits and monkeys) fed infrequently the serum cholesterol level and the incidence of atheroma are higher than in those allowed to nibble all day long. Studies of men with heart disease in Czechoslovakia showed that most of them ate less frequent meals than comparable controls. More recently both population studies and biochemical research have suggested that when a diet of the same calorie value is given either on gorging or nibbling regimens the gorgers tend to have higher blood-lipid levels and to gain more weight than the nibblers.

HARD AND SOFT WATER

The evidence from these investigations of coronary heart disease, fat metabolism, sugar, fibre and eating frequency all points in the same direction: there are good medical reasons for advising a diet similar to those believed to be natural for primitive man. A final factor is the nature of the domestic water supply. The relative merits of hard and soft water were thought to be of interest mainly to plumbers and washer-women until 1957, when a Japanese doctor first suggested that deaths from heart disease and stroke were commoner in communities with a soft-water supply than in those where the water was hard. Within a few years this link between soft water and cardiovascular disease had been confirmed in careful research studies in Britain, North America and Scandinavia.

During the 1960s it became apparent that there are other soft-water effects. Mothers in soft-water areas are more likely to give birth to babies with spina bifida, anencephaly and related congenital disorders of the brain and spine (p. 280). In addition, infant mortality is increased in soft-water areas. These possible associations are discussed in more detail in Chapter 10.

No convincing explanation has been suggested for the link between water and these apparently unrelated disorders. But for heart disease research has excluded the possibility that the excess of adult deaths from it could be due to a chance connection between the geographical distribution of soft-water supplies and, for example, adverse social conditions. A study in 1971 examined changes in death rates in those areas in England and Wales that had (for several different reasons) changed the composition of their water in the previous thirty years. Compared with the death rates from other conditions, there was a favourable effect on deaths from heart disease in the areas that had changed to a harder water supply: and conversely there was an unfavourable effect in the areas in which the water had become softer. The magnitude of this soft-water effect varies from area to area, and other factors such as race may be relevant, but in most communities a switch from hard to soft water probably increases the risk of death from cardiovascular disease by about 15 per cent – enough to account for 7,000 deaths a year in Britain in men aged between forty-five and sixty-four.

The many theoretical explanations that have been devised for the soft-water effect fall into two main classes: they either postulate a harmful constituent in soft water or suppose that hard water has some protective property. The problem is further complicated since either the harmful or the protective effect, or indeed both, could be responsible for the increased risk of heart disease, while an entirely separate factor could be responsible for the increase in the numbers of birth malformations.

The earliest explanations offered were simple deficiency theories. Hard water contains magnesium as well as calcium, and one theory was that most people in soft-water areas were suffering from mild magnesium deficiency. Rabbits fed a high-cholesterol diet low in magnesium developed atheroma more rapidly than rabbits on a high-magnesium diet: perhaps the same was true of man? As so often happens with attractive theories based on experiments on animals, large-scale research in man failed to support the magnesium/atheroma explanation. Post-mortem examination of men who had died suddenly from heart-attacks showed that if anything the men in soft-water areas had less atheroma than those from hard-water areas. The most likely explanation for this finding is that the heart-muscle of men in the soft-water group was more sensitive to a sudden diminution of its blood supply than that of the men in the hard-water group; so heart-attacks of equal severity might cause death in one area and not in the other.

Nevertheless, it remains possible that the difference in sensitivity of heart muscle is linked with the small but definite differences in the average amount of magnesium and calcium in the body which exist between communities whose water is hard and those who have soft water. The alternative possibility is that soft water may be poisonous. Most substances used in plumbing are somewhat soluble in water, though in practice this is a problem only with soft water, since the calcium salts in hard water soon form a scale on the inside of water pipes and this stops the piping being dissolved. No such scale forms with soft water, and even very small quantities of pipe metal dissolved in drinking water may have a cumulative effect. The greatest danger comes from a combination of acid, peaty soft water and lead piping, and cases of lead poisoning from this cause still occur in Britain. Doctors still do not agree on the safe level of lead in the blood, and one possible explanation for the 'soft-water factor' is chronic lead poisoning at a level far below that which produces recognizable symptoms of classical lead poisoning. Another possibility is that cadmium or zinc from galvanized water tanks or pipes may be responsible. All these toxic theories are being examined at present.

VITAMINS

Despite the claims of some health-food enthusiasts, today's average good mixed diet contains more than enough vitamins for our daily needs. Nor is there any evidence for suggestions in advertisements that vitamin tablets can give you more energy or restore youth to the middle-aged. One so-called, vitamin, vitamin E, found in wheat-germ oil has no known function in man, though the amount of the vitamin in the blood does affect the behaviour of red blood cells in laboratory tests and it has been shown to reverse sterility in rats. Claims that vitamin E can help in cases of human sterility or put back the effect of ageing have not been substantiated.

Physical illness from deficiency of vitamins may occur in malnourished communities, among food faddists and in sufferers from intestinal disorders affecting the digestion and absorption of food. Less well known are the disorders due to excess of vitamins. Too much vitamin A may lead to fatigue, sleeplessness and painful joints, while polar explorers who have eaten polar bear liver – which contains a particularly large amount of vitamin A – have developed acute poisoning.

Deficiency of vitamin A is rare in Western society since it is found in a wide variety of foods: vegetables, milk, butter, margarine, cheese, liver and fish.

Several different vitamins make up the 'B group', and B1, B2 and B3 may be considered together since deficiency of any of these individual vitamins is rare. Vitamin B1, or thiamine, is found in a wide variety of foods; pure deficiency leads eventually to beri-beri, in which there is heart failure or degeneration of the nerves, or both. Vitamin B2, or riboflavine, occurs in milk, liver and meat, eggs and vegetables; pure deficiency leads to redness and soreness of the tongue, and a rash around the nose and the corners of the mouth. The third major B vitamin, nicotinamide, is found in yeast, liver and meat, nuts and vegetables; pure deficiency leads to pellagra, with inflammation of the skin and the membranes lining the digestive system, and mental changes.

One or several of the features of vitamin B deficiency may occur in alcoholics who take little but a liquid diet. The body needs more thiamine than usual to help in the breakdown of alcohol, and so alcoholics may develop the features of early beri-beri. So faced with an alcoholic patient who has heart failure and/or loss of sensation in part of the arms and legs together with painful muscle cramps, many doctors will try the effect of an injection of mixed B vitamins – sometimes with good results. Another disease seen in some alcoholic patients affects the brain, leading to disturbances of vision and to sensory disorders. Characteristically they will tell the doctor intricate and expansive stories of what they have been doing in the last few hours, when all the time they have really been lying in the hospital bed.

Vegetarians can usually obtain all the vitamins they need from their diet, but there is one exception: strict vegetarians who take neither eggs nor milk and its products (vegans) may suffer from a deficiency of vitamin B12, or cyanocobalamin – a substance found in liver and meat which is essential for the formation of blood cells. Although various yeast products contain a little of the vitamin, it is difficult for vegetarians to obtain enough to prevent the development of anaemia, particularly during pregnancy. Such people may develop an illness which is little different from pernicious anaemia and may have to be treated with vitamin preparations; one example was Bernard Shaw, who, faced with a choice between death and modifying his principles, finally consented to have injections of liver extract. Nowadays preparations of the pure vitamin are available for injection and some may be taken by mouth.

Vitamin C, or ascorbic acid, is present in fruit and vegetables. Deficiency leads to scurvy, with mental confusion and bleeding internally and into the skin and joints. As long ago as 1753 James Lind showed that oranges and lemons rapidly cured scurvy in sailors, the traditional sufferers from the disease during long sea voyages. But it took a long time for the lesson to be learnt, particularly that people doing really hard work needed more of the vitamin than sedentary ones: the tragic end of Scott's mission to the Antarctic was due as much to the team's developing scurvy as any other factor.

Today four groups of people may develop scurvy. Firstly, babies kept on feeds of cow's milk (which contains only a quarter of the amount of vitamin C contained in human milk) without any supplements of orange juice. Secondly, mentally subnormal children, who may spit out any orange juice or fruit given them. Thirdly, patients with food fads, sometimes originating medically (as in the old-fashioned treatment of stomach ulcers, which forbade stringy vegetables and fruit with pips) and continued long after the original condition has been cured. Fourthly, people living alone – the so-called 'bachelor's scurvy'. Elderly widows and widowers often live on cups of tea and bread and butter, and not uncommonly scurvy follows a sudden shock, particularly the death of a spouse (p. 24). On the other hand, experts now no longer believe the much-publicized assertion that most old people are on the edge of scurvy. Nor is there any evidence that large doses of vitamin C can protect against the common cold. Although large doses have always been said to be harmless a recent report (admittedly in a single case) suggested that this may have caused blood-clotting in the leg veins.

Linus Pauling, the distinguished American scientist and double Nobel laureate, has attracted wide interest by his theories that very high intakes of vitamin C – up to 10 gm. daily – promote optimum health and protect against infections, especially the common cold. The theory is not accepted by official bodies in Europe or the USA: in 1974 the joint report of the British Agricultural and Medical Research Councils stated that 'there is very little sound evidence to support this view and in fact there is some reason to suspect that high intakes could be harmful'. Several attempts have been made to test the theory in scientific trials in which some volunteers took vitamin C and others took dummy tablets of identical appearance. None of these trials showed any convincing benefit from the vitamin C in reducing the number or severity of colds.

Vitamin D, or calciferol, is obtained in two ways: from milk, liver and eggs; and made by the body itself in the skin under the influence of sunlight. Lack of vitamin D means that insufficient calcium is absorbed from the intestines; eventually the bones become weakened, leading to rickets in children and to osteomalacia in pregnant women. Although these conditions became particularly prevalent in Britain in the industrial revolution, with its poor diet and smoky atmosphere shutting out the sunlight, they still occur even with today's increased prosperity and clean air – and with no other vitamin are so many people at risk of having too little. Unfortunately there is also a risk in adding the vitamin to food, because too much of it may endanger health. Four classes of people need vitamin D supplements (given, say, as cod-liver-oil capsules): babies, pregnant women, the elderly house-bounds and many immigrants. Surveys of immigrant communities have shown that as many as two fifths of the children and one fifth of the adults have some evidence of vitamin D deficiency. The dark skin of many immigrants (particularly Indians and Pakistanis) means that sunlight has a less stimulating effect on the skin's production of vitamin D than in a lighter-skinned person – and anyway traditionally many immigrants spend most of their leisure indoors. Another factor is that a chemical in the chappatis, which many immigrants eat every day, may prevent calcium being absorbed in the intestines. Certainly the recurrence of rickets in many of our Northern towns – such as Glasgow, Manchester and Rochdale – has caused much concern to the medical authorities there.

Finally, vitamin K, which is essential for the normal process of blood-clotting after an injury, occurs in a wide range of vegetables and is also formed within the intestines by bacteria present there. Deficiency occurs only in persons suffering from disease of the liver or intestines.

Chapter 3

FOOD POISONING

THE history of food poisoning goes back to biblical times, for the prohibition laid on the Jews against eating pork and drinking milk probably had its origin in the likelihood that these foods could spread disease. Although several serious diseases (such as poliomyelitis or hepatitis) may be spread by infected food or water, the term 'food poisoning' usually means an illness coming on suddenly after eating contaminated food. There are three main types of food poisoning – caused by bacteria or their poisonous toxins; plants and animals; and chemicals. Food-poisoning symptoms develop within hours and are usually stomach pains, diarrhoea and sickness. Occasionally more serious complications may develop, such as paralysis and double vision or temporary blindness.

BACTERIAL POISONING

Three main types of bacteria are implicated in the vast majority of cases of bacterial food poisoning: salmonellae, staphylococci and clostridia. The first causes illness by direct infection of the digestive system; the latter two involve toxins produced by the bacteria.

Official food-poisoning statistics are only the tip of the iceberg, for relatively few incidents are notified. But such figures as we have indicate that 80–90 per cent of incidents can be traced to contaminated meat or poultry, and that two thirds of the identified cases are caused by salmonellae. The salmonellae are minute rod-shaped bacteria which cause enteric fever (typhoid and paratyphoid fever: see p. 75) and many less severe infections that are usually grouped as 'salmonellosis'. These salmonellae are sometimes present in the intestines of men, animals and birds, and are transmitted by contamination of food and drink with faeces. Animals – cattle, pigs and particularly chickens – form a reservoir for salmonellae, which they usually get from contaminated feeding stuffs, particularly fish meal. In 1971 official tests showed that 23 per cent of samples of fish meal and bone meal contained salmonellae. When animals are slaughtered and processed under conditions which allow bacteria to multiply there is always a risk of infection. Proper cooking should kill bacteria, but is often not thorough enough, and in any case there is a risk to the people handling the raw food – slaughterers, butchers and housewives. Food-handlers may have a brief attack of salmonellosis and then become carriers – symptomless excreters of the micro-organisms in faeces and urine – and hence unwittingly liable to spread the infection. Milk which is not pasteurized may also be contaminated by salmonellae, and transmit infection.

In a typical outbreak of salmonellosis meat or poultry has been cooked in such a way that not all the bacteria have been killed. The meat is not eaten immediately but stored at room temperature for a day or so. Storage at any temperature above 4°C. (that of a refrigerator) allows any surviving bacteria to multiply sufficiently to produce food poisoning when the food is eaten. Alternatively, all the bacteria in the food may have been killed by adequate cooking, but it may then become contaminated again by salmonellae left from raw food on the kitchen working surfaces and pots and pans; again, storage at room temperature allows these germs to multiply.

Victims of salmonellosis usually develop a sudden attack of sickness and diarrhoea within twelve hours of eating the contaminated food. Medical detective work shows that the outbreak usually follows one of three patterns. Firstly, it may affect a hospital or residential home over a long period, and be difficult to trace, though one of the staff or a patient who is a carrier may eventually be identified as the source. Secondly, a single explosive outbreak may result when contaminated food is eaten at a single meal, such as a dinner or a wedding reception. Thirdly, a series of widely distributed outbreaks may eventually be traced back to a single source such as a central butchery.

Fortunately salmonellosis is usually only a brief episode: if the patient goes to bed for a day or so, he recovers rapidly. Antibiotics or admission to hospital are rarely necessary, but any food-handler should get a check-up before he returns to work to make sure he has not become a carrier of the germ.

Staphylococci are minute, round bacteria which characteristically grow microscopically in clumps looking something like a bunch of grapes. They are present all over the body surface and inside the mouth and nose. Many types of staphylococci are harmless, but others cause boils or abscesses. Some types can produce a toxin when they grow on foods such as meat. As with salmonellosis, food poisoning due to staphylococcal toxin is usually associated with eating precooked meat that has been stored at room temperature for a day or two. But in this case the bacteria are usually introduced when the food is sliced immediately after cooking, by a food-handler who is carrying staphylococci on the skin or the nose or who has a cut or septic spot. Even careful hand-washing may not get rid of the bacteria, which stick closely to the skin and lodge in crevices on the body surface. Storage of the food at room temperature then allows the staphylococci to multiply and produce toxin. Usually sickness and pain come on suddenly an hour or two after eating meat or dairy products. The latter may be contaminated in the same way as meat, or the bacteria may have come from a cow or goat with mastitis, a staphylococcal infection of the udder. Most people recover within a few hours, but sometimes they are severely prostrated – and may even die.

Clostridia are minute, rod-shaped bacteria which include the types causing tetanus, gas-gangrene and botulism (see p. 65). *Clostridium welchii*, which produces a toxin causing some kinds of food poisoning, is widespread in the environment, including dust, and is often present in raw meat. A particular risk here is that clostridia can form spores which resist the heat of cooking and then germinate once the food has cooled to room temperature. If the food is not stored in a refrigerator the bacteria can multiply rapidly and produce the powerful toxin. Moreover, some strains of clostridia may survive fairly high temperatures (90°C.), levels which quite possibly are not reached inside a chicken carcass during cooking. Cross-contamination from surfaces used for preparing uncooked meat is another possible route of infection.

Clostridial food poisoning is also seen usually after eating meat which has been cooked the day before and not refrigerated overnight. People develop symptoms twelve to twenty-four hours after the meal, usually severe diarrhoea and abdominal pain. Almost always they recover unless they are old and/or run down. This is the typical 'mild' form of clostridial food poisoning. Another form, which is due to a different strain of the germ, is much more serious and is often fatal, because it causes extensive damage to the intestines. It is associated with eating home-canned meat and has been seen chiefly in Germany.

None of these bacteria produce any detectable changes in the food they contaminate, so that this type of food poisoning means a strict code for handling food. By law food shops are not allowed to sell animal foods as well unless these are in a sealed container. Food handlers may not work if they have a cut or septic spot on their skin and they must wear 'clean and washable' clothing; they are also required to keep their instruments and working surfaces clean.

Deep-frozen food should be thawed and cooked for long enough: chickens, for example, should thaw for at least eight hours at room temperature and then be cooked at 190–204°C. for thirty minutes per pound. Meat should be cooked in joints not heavier than 6 lb. to ensure that sufficient heat can penetrate into the centre.

To overcome the problems facing all institutional cooking, food is best served hot as soon as it is ready; it should be cut immediately without touching it by hand, and kept at a temperature above 60°C. until needed. If cold sliced meat is required, it should be sliced immediately after cooking; placed in metal trays to cool rapidly; and refrigerated within an hour. The same working surfaces should not be used for slicing cooked meat as for raw meat.

The problem of salmonellosis could also be tackled in another way – at the probable principal source of the infection – by insisting that bone and fish meal used as animal feedstuffs should be treated before distribution. In Denmark, where such treatment is enforced by law, research has shown that salmonellae were present in only 0·3 per cent of samples of meal, compared with 23 per cent of British samples. Today the incidence of salmonellosis is falling in Denmark whereas it is rising in Britain. As a leading article in the *Lancet* remarked, 'It is a strange reflection on industry and public health alike that knowingly we allow animals to eat salmonellae in foods which they, in turn, pass back in the food they supply. Perhaps the time has come for legislation, in Britain, as in Denmark.'

Detective work

In most cases the person with bacterial food poisoning has much the same symptoms whatever the type of germ causing it, so that the precise nature of the infection is usually of interest only to the bacteriologist. But sometimes the laboratory and epidemiological investigations needed to unravel the cause and its source have all the fascination of a good crime story. Such a case was an incident affecting twelve people who had been on a flight from Bangkok to London. Detective work showed that all of the passengers had been infected with a bacterium known as *Vibrio parahaemolyticus* (the same general type as that causing cholera) and had also eaten a crab cocktail prepared for the airline in Bangkok. This bacterium, which is frequently found in food in summer in Japan and the Far East, was then isolated from samples of raw crab claws (which had been immediately flown over from Bangkok), and also from the *hors d'œuvres* served during the flight.

Nearer home, much the same sort of painstaking work was needed to find out the cause of several outbreaks of food poisoning in diners in a Chinese restaurant. All of these had eaten fried rice, whereas their table companions who had chosen boiled rice had remained perfectly well. Laboratory tests on the rice showed that it contained large numbers of the micro-organism *Bacillus cereus*, and the same bacterium was also isolated from many of the patients. *Bacillus cereus* is normally present in rice, but does little harm since it is killed by cooking. The next step in the British outbreak was to discover exactly how this particular Chinese restaurant prepared its fried rice. This was usually based on the leftover portions of boiled rice, which were allowed to remain by the warm stove so that they could be fried straight away. Sometimes, in fact, stale boiled rice was left at room temperature over the weekend before being fried at Monday lunchtime. All this meant that this outbreak had almost certainly occurred as follows. Boiling had killed the actual germs in the rice, but not the spores, which can withstand much higher temperatures. So in the next few hours the warm surroundings of the kitchen enabled the spores to germinate, forming large numbers of *Bacillus cereus* again and also a mild toxin, which had then produced food poisoning. The obvious moral is not to keep boiled rice around at room temperature at all, but, since the grains stick together if it is kept in a refrigerator, to discard it altogether if it is not used at that meal.

A much more serious illness associated with bacterial spores is botulism, due to a powerful toxin produced by the organism *Clostridium botulinum*. The spores of this germ are present widely throughout soil, lakeshore mud and seaside sand. They are not killed by boiling but only by a temperature of at least 120°C. for thirty minutes or more. When oxygen is not present, the spores present in food can germinate into the parent germ, *Clostridium botulinum*, and at the same time produce one of the most lethal poisons known. (According to the *Guinness Book of Records* 410 grammes would kill the entire human population of the world.) This may occur during home-canning or bottling, particularly if the food is not acid enough to prevent the spores from germinating, such as string beans, peas, corn and spinach. As well as fruit and vegetables, smoke-cured and salt-cured meat and fish have also caused several outbreaks of botulism and, though the food may seem obviously 'off', this is not always so and minor changes in taste may be disguised by the strong flavour of the food.

Characteristically the illness starts within twelve to thirty-six hours of eating the food: the patient becomes giddy, sees double and develops muscle weakness and difficulty in swallowing and breathing. In most outbreaks between 30 and 100 per cent of those affected have died. Patients are treated with injections of an antitoxin specific to whichever of the six different types of the germ has caused the illness, and by treating the main symptoms, such as using an artificial respirator to help breathing difficulties.

Fortunately in Britain botulism is rare because our commercial canners have high standards, home-canning is actively discouraged, and we do not eat much smoked fish. In fact, the last major outbreak in this country occurred in August 1922, when all eight members of a fishing party on Loch Maree died after eating sandwiches made of potted wild duck paste. There were smaller outbreaks in 1947 and 1955.

Occasional outbreaks of botulism still occur on the Continent of Europe and in the USA. In 1971, for example, a man in New York died after eating cold vichyssoise soup from a tin marketed by a commercial firm. Routine checks by another large firm on their soups then showed that some tins contained the botulinus germ; people who had bought them were asked to throw them away and claim a refund.

PLANT POISONING

Over 200 varieties of plants are said to be poisonous to man, but fortunately even the so-called poisonous plants rarely cause more than a few mild symptoms. Less than 10 per cent of children seen in hospital casualty departments for poisoning have swallowed seeds, berries or leaves, compared with 66 per cent who have taken medicines and 20 per cent who have drunk household fluids. So in practice serious poisoning from plants usually arise from mistaking the particular plant for another edible one. Among the most serious are the nightshades, the death-cap and fly agaric mushrooms and monkshood. The berries of deadly nightshade may be mistaken for blackberries; they contain belladonna, or atropine, which causes dryness of the skin, fever, delirium and coma – a condition summed up by two American child specialists as 'hot as a hare, blind as a bat, dry as a bone, red as a beet and mad as a hen'. There is no specific treatment for atropine poisoning and it may end fatally. Monkshood, which may be mistaken for horse-radish, contains aconitine, which gives rise to pricking sensations under the skin (called 'formication') and paralysis of breathing. The death-cap mushroom, *Amanita phalloides*, is virtually the only mushroom which may kill; expert knowledge is needed to distinguish it from the edible mushroom and the only safeguard is to eat those bought in shops. About 30 per cent of those who eat *Amanita phalloides* in mistake for the edible mushroom die from its effects, and throughout the world several hundred people are said to be killed by it every year. *Amanita phalloides* produces one of the most powerful poisons known; poisoning develops between four and twenty-four hours after eating only one or two mushrooms, with abdominal pain, vomiting and diarrhoea. A few days later signs of liver and kidney failure appear, and these complications are often lethal. Poisoning by *Amanita muscaria*, the fly agaric, is less serious and develops earlier, after two hours. Characteristically people become confused and mildly drunk; and this species was used deliberately by Siberian peasants to relieve the unpleasantness of their lives and possibly also as 'the sacred mushroom' by some religious sects. Other symptoms of poisoning include diarrhoea and vomiting, but usually the outlook is good.

Although it has not been seen in Britain since 1928, and the last outbreak occurred in France in 1951, ergot poisoning is still of interest because of its role in causing 'St Anthony's fire' – an epidemic disease common in tenth- and eleventh-century Europe, in which people developed convulsions, hallucinations and dancing mania. The fire of the condition's name was the intolerable burning pain in the limbs, and when subsequently these became blackened through the onset of gangrene, they were likened to charcoal. Sufferers were treated at houses devoted to the Order of St Anthony, and the walls of these hospitals were painted a symbolic red or flame colour.

The cause of St Anthony's fire was contamination of grain, particularly rye, with fungus *Claviceps purpurea*, which tends to occur after a wet sowing and a wet summer. Bread made from this so-called 'smutty' rye often contains ergot, which produces complex effects on the body but particularly spasm of the blood vessels. At first this gives rise to tingling and pricking sensations and pain in the limbs, but if the person goes on eating ergot, gangrene may develop, together with other features such as painful muscles, seizures and mental changes. It should be easy for the farmer and the miller to recognize infected grain, since the ergot particles are larger and darker. Even so, in 1951 modern methods of supervision and distribution did not prevent a severe outbreak of ergotism in France: 200 of the 4,000 inhabitants of the Provençal village of Pont St Esprit developed the condition, with delirium and hallucinations; old and young were reported as running frantic in the streets, while many others lay writhing and screaming on their beds; at least four people died. Possibly this outbreak was due to LSD, which this type of fungus may also produce.

Before this there had been a large outbreak in Russia during 1926–7, affecting over 10,000 people. Our immunity to the disease in Britain is largely due to our national preference for wheat rather than rye bread and not necessarily to the high quality of rye grown in this country – as was shown in 1928, when an outbreak of ergotism affected 200 Jewish refugees from Central Europe who were living in Manchester: they had eaten ergot-infected bread which had been made from diseased rye harvested in Yorkshire.

Plant products may cause another type of food poisoning that still occurs, commonly in the USA and Canada and occasionally in Britain: that is, 'musselling', or shellfish poisoning. Bivalve shellfish, such as mussels, oysters, cockles and scallops, feed on plankton (in particular a dinoflagellate *Gonyaulax tamarensis*). Some species of this are red-coloured and contain a toxin, so-called saxitoxin, which is concentrated by the bivalves – though these themselves are unaffected by it. When such shellfish are eaten poisoning develops within half an hour. The main symptoms are tingling in the fingers, hands and mouth, weakness and a peculiar sensation of floating; occasionally people die from paralysis of breathing. Sea-water often contains small quantities of plankton that produce toxin but there are not enough of them to cause poisoning. Occasionally the number of algae rises dangerously and may be seen as a 'red tide' in the sea. For this reason experts regularly monitor shellfish for their toxin content; if this is too high, they forbid commercial fishing and warn the public of the dangers of collecting and eating them.

The role of other fungi in causing human disease is less certain. By itself, ordinary mould is fairly harmless, though it is an indication that food has been kept under conditions which could also encourage the growth of harmful bacteria. But one mould that has caused concern is *Aspergillus flavus,* which produces substances known as aflatoxins. In the early 1960s these were found to have caused an outbreak of fatal liver damage in turkeys given feeds of contaminated groundnuts. Research then showed that not only did aflatoxins seriously damage the liver in many animal species, but that the surviving animals were particularly liable to develop liver cancer. The obvious question then was whether aflatoxins played any part in human liver cancer, particularly since this disease is much commoner in African countries than in the West. Subsequently aflatoxins were detected in 40 per cent of Ugandan foods, particularly in groundnuts, which are a staple food in that country. The suggestion of an aflatoxin–cancer link seemed to be reinforced when it was also found that the poorest tribes (which are particularly likely to eat mouldy foods) have the highest incidence of liver cancer. Most recently three separate surveys have shown that the amount of liver cancer in a community ties in very closely with the amounts of aflatoxin in the food eaten. In Thailand the inhabitants of one province eat food with a higher than average aflatoxin content, and they have three times as much liver cancer as other provinces. Similar results were found in Kenya; while in Mozambique there is one district where the aflatoxin content of the food is the highest in the world: so is the incidence of liver cancer.

Aflatoxins have also been incriminated in a rare disorder (Reye's syndrome), in which small children lose consciousness due to a combination of brain and liver disturbances. Almost certainly one cause of this syndrome – found in the Pacific, including New Zealand, more often than in Europe – is due to aflatoxins formed in contaminated rice.

CHEMICALS

Several chemicals present in food may cause poisoning. The element cadmium tends to accumulate in the body with age, from sources such as drinking water, flour, coffee and tea, vegetables and cigarettes. This amount does not apparently harm health, but acute food poisoning may arise when old-fashioned cooking pots lined with cadmium are used to prepare acid food. The acid releases cadmium and often antimony as well into the food. People may develop acute poisoning, with the usual symptoms, within fifteen to forty-five minutes of eating the contaminated food, but normally they recover rapidly. In Japan long-standing heavy industrial pollution by cadmium of the drinking water and of the crops along the Jintsu river was said to be responsible for 'itai-itai', or 'ouch-ouch' disease (p. 205).

In this country the government is monitoring cadmium levels in food and a recent report stated that there was no hazard to the average consumer. Another report, published at the same time, came to the same conclusion about the hazard of mercury compounds in food. This had come into the limelight when tuna fish was found to contain some inorganic mercury (p. 205) and was emphasized by the Minimata Bay disaster (p. 204) of serious methyl-mercury poisoning. Methyl-mercury compounds are also used as seed dressings, and people have been poisoned from eating pork from pigs fed on treated grain. In Iraq in 1971 many hundreds of people died and several thousands developed serious brain damage from eating grain which had been dressed with methyl-mercury after the sowing season.

People often ask what cooking pots and pans are safe to use. Aluminium and stainless steel pans are quite inert and no metal passes into the food. Copper pans seem to be safe, particularly if they are lined by tin, which prevents copper passing into the food. If the tinned surface is lost, however, acid food may rapidly dissolve the copper and cause food poisoning; one such outbreak was associated with cooking stewed apples. Similarly, fruit juices may occasionally dissolve the tin in tin cans and produce acute poisoning. The rate of dissolving tin from cans is probably faster if nitrates are present in the product.

A curiosity which has caused several episodes of food poisoning is copper sulphate, produced in gas-heated water boilers. A typical outbreak was reported from Bolton, where twenty workmen drank early-morning tea made from water heated in a geyser and soon afterwards developed diarrhoea and sickness. Sulphur present in the gas fumes was found to have corroded the copper lid of the geyser, producing copper sulphate, and tests on samples of tea made from this geyser contained fifteen times the acceptable amount of copper.

Although this is not strictly food poisoning, young children may develop lead poisoning from chewing paint or eating soil contaminated with lead (pica). This is discussed on p. 196.

FOOD ADDITIVES

Over 20,000 food additives are now known, and everyone in Britain eats about 3 lb. of them every year. Additives are non-nutritive substances added intentionally to food to improve its appearance, flavour, texture or storage, but despite much research we still know comparatively little about whether most of these affect our health. Occasionally a substance has been banned because research has shown that it may harm animals. Even so, different animal species react differently to different substances, and large quantities of a particular substance are usually employed in research tests. Hence the two main questions are whether the minute quantities taken occasionally by man are harmful, and what action, if any, should be taken. Obviously, also, any decision will depend on the possible risk and what the substance is used for. A colouring agent, for example, can be discarded and replaced by something less harmful, whereas this may not be possible or desirable with an artificial sweetener. Recently, the red-colouring agent used in many different foods, Ponceau XX, was withdrawn after research had shown that rats fed large quantities developed liver tumours. In the USA the so-called Delaney clause makes it illegal to add anything to food that induces cancer in animals. Bladder cancer is now known to be commoner in rats fed high concentrations of saccharin, and at one time it seemed that it would be banned, as cyclamates have been. The whole debate in the case of cyclamates illustrates how difficult it is to apply laboratory findings to man.

Several years ago large doses of cyclamates given to hamsters were found to have seriously damaged the heart and the kidneys. Further research showed that rats given cyclamates developed bladder tumours – a finding which eventually led to this artificial sweetening agent being banned by several countries, including the USA, Sweden and Britain. But at the time it was pointed out how illogical such a ban was: many people had taken moderate quantities of cyclamates for years without ill-effect; the experimental dose used had been very large; only some species of animal had reacted in this way, and on the basis of abnormal results produced in some animals we should have had to forgo two valuable drugs introduced before such tests had been routine – thiouracil and penicillin. Cyclamates had helped to make life tolerable for many people whose diet had had to be carefully restricted, such as diabetics and the obese on a weight-reducing diet, and on present knowledge the risks of obesity are much higher than those of cyclamates.

Further research should show whether this particular ban was justified, but undoubtedly any agent that can cause cancer in animals must be evaluated very carefully for its safety. This is now being done for nitrates, which for years have been used for preserving fish such as salmon and herring, as well as meat such as ham and bacon, and some cheeses. When food is stored, nitrosamines may be produced – substances which readily cause cancer in animals at very low dosage levels. Nitrates also occur naturally in some foods, such as spinach, and they may be formed in some parts of the body from nitrates present in drinking water or food.

Nitrosamines have also been found in African native beer and spirits and it has been suggested that these may be linked with the commonness of cancer of the oesophagus in that continent, which has already been statistically associated with drinking locally produced spirits. The low intake of protein in Africa may also enhance the effect of nitrosamines, but in Western countries experts believe that nitros-amines have no important role in causing cancer. The same is true of the small quantities of known cancer-producing substances produced by cooking, such as in grilling meat. Almost certainly these substances pass through the intestines and are not absorbed. Cooking probably also destroys the traces of antibiotics and hormones present in meat from animals given them to increase their growth.

INSECTICIDES

A few substances, however, are not destroyed by cooking or in the body, and in fact may accumulate there; for instance, insecticides such as DDT (dicophane), BHC (benzene hexa-chloride) and dieldrin in the body-fat stores. For many years these have been widely used for controlling pests, particularly in the tropics, where they are estimated to have saved ten million lives from malaria alone. Because they are used extensively in agriculture they find their way into food-stuffs, mainly as animal fats, and some of this is laid down in human fat stores. In animals given insecticides followed by an insecticide-free diet it takes several years before the level of insecticides stored in fat is halved. Insecticides cross the placenta from the mother to the unborn baby, which starts off life with some of them in its body-fat; breast milk, and to a lesser extent cows' milk, also contains insecticides.

The levels of BHC and dieldrin in human fat are roughly similar throughout the world, but that of DDT varies con-siderably with the individual country concerned, people in America having twice and those of India fifteen times the average in Britain. Moreover, although nobody has shown that people are harmed by persistent insecticides, most of us have welcomed recent evidence that levels of insecticide in human fat have fallen progressively in those countries which have restricted their use in the last ten years.

All this means that evaluation of food hazards is in its infancy and depends mostly on continuous surveillance and testing programmes by official bodies. Even so, the importance of anecdotal reports which pinpoint a particular hazard should not be underestimated. Such a report led to the discovery of the 'Chinese restaurant syndrome' or 'Kwok's Quease'. In this, susceptible people developed burning or tightening feelings in their necks, arms and chests about twenty minutes after eating at Chinese restaurants. The condition, which usually passed off after forty-five minutes, was found to be due to large quantities of monosodium glutamate, a substance used in some Chinese restaurants to enhance the flavour of the food. Similarly, nitrates have been shown to be the cause of 'hot-dog' headache, which occurs in some people after eating sausages or cured meat containing nitrate as a preservative. Some people who are liable to migraine find that their headaches are brought on by certain foods, including chocolate, cheese, citrus fruits and alcohol; one of the substances responsible may be tyrosine present in the food. Finally, the importance of simple medical detective work has recently been emphasized by a report from a Swedish skin specialist, who has shown that a colouring agent widely used in manufactured food may be responsible for some skin conditions such as eczema.

EPIDEMIC INFECTIONS

Two main groups of major infections are transmitted by food: those when the food becomes contaminated by handling during preparation (hand-to-mouth spread), and those when the raw food is infected itself or contaminated before it is handled (as by worm eggs).

Typhoid fever, due to infection with the germ *Salmonella typhi*, is the most serious illness caused by the *salmonella* group of bacteria. The other type of enteric fever, paratyphoid fever, due to infection with *Salmonella paratyphi* A or B, is much milder and rarely fatal. Unlike the other 1,000 or so salmonellae, those causing enteric fever infect only man and not animals. Thus the reservoir of enteric fever is usually a carrier, somebody who has recovered from the infection but goes on excreting the bacteria in the urine and faeces, often because of hidden infection in the gall-bladder or bone-marrow. Roughly one in every 100,000 people in Britain is a carrier of enteric, but carriers are of little risk to the public if they keep to strict personal hygiene and do not handle food. If this hygiene breaks down or if the carrier is unrecognized an outbreak of enteric fever may occur.

Other methods of spread of typhoid or paratyphoid include contaminated water or food, since the bacteria can survive for weeks in water, food or sewage. Contamination of the reservoir supplying Croydon was responsible for the 1937 outbreak in the borough (344 cases; 43 deaths). The Aberdeen epidemic of 1964 (507 cases; no deaths) is thought to have originated from a can of corned beef which had been contaminated by sewage present in a South American river in which the cans had been cooled. Similarly, sporadic cases of typhoid have been traced to oysters growing in contaminated estuaries. Most of the cases of enteric fever seen in Britain, however, do not occur in epidemics but sporadically, being acquired abroad on holiday (p. 129) or in immigrants who subsequently come here.

Apart from the characteristic fever in typhoid, there is severe prostration, cough and bronchitis, rash, and enlargement of the body's lymphoid tissue, including the liver, spleen and lymph nodes. Because this enlargement affects the lymphoid tissue of the intestine it may lead to two of the main fatal complications of typhoid: severe bleeding or perforation of the intestine.

Although no outbreak has occurred in Britain since 1896, cholera flourished here for sixty years in the nineteenth century. Its disappearance reflects the facts that cholera is mainly transmitted by drinking water contaminated by sewage – and also that the disease requires a malnourished population in which to take root. Today the occasional case of cholera seen in Britain has been acquired by travel abroad (p. 128).

Dysentery is an illness in which the patient develops diarrhoea, pain in the abdomen, and blood and pus in the faeces. It may be due either to bacteria (bacillary dysentery) or to larger single-celled organisms called amoebae (amoebic dysentery). In the first type over 95 per cent of cases are due to a germ called *Shigella sonnei*, and traditionally the illness is associated with overcrowding. At one time an epidemic scourge of armies, today bacillary dysentery tends to be endemic, or persistent, and to affect younger people – particularly children in nurseries, primary schools, and institutions for the mentally retarded. It may spread in water or food, but more commonly the route is by person-to-person contact or by infection from objects that the child has touched. These objects, or fomites, can play an important part in its spread because, unlike typhoid fever and cholera, only a few germs are needed to transmit bacillary dysentery; moreover, under the right conditions, *Shigella sonnei* can survive for several weeks. Adults usually get the infection from a child with dysentery, which is one of the few infections transmitted by handling a lavatory seat, since this is readily splashed by infected material during flushing.

The link between bacillary dysentery and overcrowding explains one of its paradoxical features: it is the one major intestinal infection which is commoner in winter than in summer. One unexplained feature, however, is why its prevalence apparently varies so much, following a sine-wave pattern over the years. Thus dysentery was common in the late 1930s and early 1940s; then its incidence fell until 1949, when it suddenly rose again; and another definite fall has occurred in the early 1970s. This seems to be a true rise and fall and one not due to fashions in notification of the disease. The disease itself may be very mild, with only slight diarrhoea, or even none at all.

Amoebic dysentery is transmitted by food or water contaminated by faeces containing cysts of the amoeba *Entamoeba histolytica*. These cysts hatch out in the intestine and sometimes invade its wall, forming abscesses; occasionally the infection may spread to the liver or lung, or even the brain. Actual dysentery occurs in only about a third of cases, usually in epidemics due to contaminated water. More often, people are infected via food-handlers and complain of a vague, prolonged illness with abdominal pain, lethargy and bodily aches; hence when amoebae are present somewhere in the body the condition is usually called amoebiasis. Amoebiasis is more common (and often more severe) in the tropics, but is not uncommon in temperate climates, and in Britain about 5 per cent of the population carries *Entamoeba histolytica* in the intestine, though usually the infection does not spread elsewhere in the body.

Another of the single-celled organisms (or protozoa) that may infect the intestines, in the tropics or temperate zones, is *Giardia lamblia*. Like *Entamoeba histolytica*, this organism usually reaches the intestine as cysts in contaminated food. But, unlike amoebiasis, giardiasis is almost invariably mild, and *Giardia lamblia* may be a chance finding on microscopic examination of the faeces, particularly in children. In adults, on the other hand, a sudden heavy primary infection may produce severe diarrhoea and abdominal pain, or may resemble appendicitis. Such an outbreak was reported in 1971 in a group of Swedish students who spent a week at a Leningrad hotel (giardiasis is said to be common in the USSR); no fewer than thirty out of the thirty-eight developed symptoms four to seven days later, with frequent diarrhoea, abdominal pain and a bloated feeling. These symptoms persisted for up to three weeks, when treatment was started.

WORMS AND FLUKES

A similar wide variation in symptoms is found when several types of worms lodge in the intestine (such as whipworm, roundworm and pinworm). Because symptoms may often be absent, the term 'infestation' is frequently used rather than 'infection'. Whether a person develops symptoms or not seems to depend on age, nutritional state and the heaviness of the infestation, as well as whether the worms remain confined to the intestine or move elsewhere in the body. Many of these worms are transmitted by food that has been manured with human faeces, and so this type of infestation is commoner in poor, rural areas than in urban ones.

One worm that hits the British headlines occasionally is the liver-fluke, or flatworm, *Fasciola hepatica*, which has caused a few episodes of illness associated with eating wild watercress. The fluke has a complicated life-cycle involving two hosts, snails and, normally, sheep and cattle. Eggs released from snails become encysted on near-by waterside plants; if these are eaten by cattle or men, they hatch out into flukes in the intestines, and when these are six weeks old they travel to the liver and enter the bile ducts. During this stage patients may develop fever, feel ill and lose weight, and have pain over the liver and generalized itching; often, however, the symptoms are rather vague. Even though liver-flukes are common in sheep and cattle – and represent a serious economic drain on the farmer – fewer than 100 cases of human fascioliasis have been reported. It is quite probable that some cases are totally unrecognized but the explanation for the rarity of the human disease seems to be that only a wet summer produces enough snails to ensure that the egg cysts are sufficiently widely distributed. But there is little risk of infection with liver-fluke if the person eats only watercress grown under supervised conditions.

Perhaps the best-known type of worm is the tapeworm. Some tapeworms live partly in the human intestine and the remainder of their lives in the muscles of cattle and pigs. The life-cycle starts in the latter when they eat earth contaminated with human faeces containing worm eggs, and human infestation occurs by eating inadequately cooked contaminated meat. Once in the human intestine the cysts hatch out and grow into adult worms, which may reach a length of twenty feet. In well-nourished people these worms usually do little harm, causing only vague indigestion or no symptoms at all. Rarely, a much more serious illness may occur when a person eats the eggs of the pork tapeworm (or more rarely the beef tapeworm) in contaminated food or soil. The eggs hatch out in the intestine and several days later the larvae migrate via the bloodstream all over the body – to the skin, muscles, brain, eye, heart and lungs. Once the larvae die, the body tissues react to wall them off from surrounding tissues, and in the brain these resulting masses may cause epilepsy.

Inspection of pork and beef, together with adequate cooking, would eliminate these infestations, which are relatively uncommon in most developed countries. But infestation with another tapeworm – the fish tapeworm (*Diphyllobothrium latum*) – though not seen in Britain, is common elsewhere, particularly in regions where raw fish is eaten regularly, such as Scandinavia, the USSR, USA and Japan. This is the largest tapeworm, growing to a length of thirty feet or more, and it may cause serious anaemia by depriving its host of vitamin B_{12} (p. 56) which is needed for the formation of red blood cells.

Another type of worm, a roundworm called *Trichinella spiralis*, may occur in pork and infect man if he eats it uncooked or partially cooked. Unlike the tapeworm, this roundworm spends its whole life in one host, which may be of a variety of species, including man, pigs, bears, rats, cats and dogs. The particular feature of this worm is that its larvae always migrate round the body, producing a fairly severe illness with fever, muscle pains and swelling around the eyes. Sufficient larvae may also form cysts in the brain or heart to damage them seriously. Even so, the larvae are too small to be visible to the naked eye, so that contaminated pork is not detected by routine meat inspection, though adequate cooking will kill the larvae. Surprisingly, many people still eat ordinary sausages without cooking them at all, and inquiries during typical outbreaks of trichiniasis in the Midlands in the war showed that 22 per cent of patients had done this at some time or other, often using sausage-meat to make a paste for sandwiches. Nevertheless, trichiniasis seems to have become much less common since a law making it illegal to feed pigs uncooked garbage came into force. Various exotic ways of acquiring the disease have been reported, including from partially cooked bear or walrus meat, from cheap steak *tartare* that had been adulterated with raw pork, and contamination from an unwashed meat-grinding machine that had previously been used for mincing pork.

OTHER INFECTIONS

Food may simply be infected by bacteria or worms rather than contaminated by a food handler, the two main items being meat and dairy products. At one time tuberculosis was the commonest serious hazard of raw milk or its products from an infected herd: these caused at least one in every ten cases of tuberculosis in Britain. The risk has been largely abolished, firstly, by pasteurization – killing the tuberculosis germs by keeping the milk at 70°C. for half an hour – and more recently by tuberculin testing of cattle. But testing relates only to tuberculosis, and there is still one hazard in drinking unpasteurized TT milk: brucellosis. This illness, caused by the bacterium *Brucella abortus*, is known as undulant or abortus fever, and is closely related to Malta or Mediterranean fever. The bacteria cause contagious abortion in cattle (although some infected animals may be apparently healthy), which then pass the germs into their milk. Human infection is a hazard of one's occupation (affecting farmers and veterinary surgeons) and of drinking unpasteurized milk or its products such as cream and cheese. Something between a few hundred and 1,000 people are affected in Britain every year, about one third of them being occupational in origin. The features of brucellosis are usually very vague – so vague that patients are often labelled by their doctors as neurotic. But traditionally brucellosis starts with an acute illness, with fever, heavy sweating, generalized aches and pains, and pains in the joints. This may last for two or three weeks and then recur after similar intervals for three to six months. Patients with the chronic disease are weak, extremely lethargic and irritable, and have headaches and occasional pains in the joints.

Treatment with antibiotics is effective, but has to be prolonged. Even so, brucellosis is entirely preventable today much as milk-borne tuberculosis has been for the past twenty years. Pasteurization kills the brucella organisms, and so a person is safe in drinking treated milk. But, although non-pasteurized milk is labelled 'untreated', cream is not – and so may cause infection. Other countries have carried through vigorous programmes of eradication by slaughtering affected herds and compensating the farmers: the Scandinavian countries and Western Germany are now all free of this unpleasant disease, while others are making rapid progress. In Britain a voluntary eradication programme was started in 1971, but this will take an estimated ten to fifteen years to complete.

Food may also become contaminated by viruses, particularly enteroviruses, a large group made up of several subgroups, including polioviruses and the so-called Coxsackie and Echoviruses. The first of these causes poliomyelitis, which since immunization was introduced in Western countries is now seen mainly in older people, who have not been immunized and catch it aboard, and in the developing countries. The second and third subgroups of these viruses cause various diseases ranging from an illness like the common cold, or a feverish illness with diarrhoea and vomiting, to serious meningitis or heart disease in infants.

Another illness now known to be due to a virus and transmitted by contaminated food or water is infectious hepatitis, one type of acute inflammation of the liver. The severity of the illness varies, but a feeling of being off-colour, loss of appetite and nausea are common, and jaundice may occur, though not in every case. Sporadic masked and obvious cases occur frequently, and epidemics may affect institutions or members of the armed forces. Infectious hepatitis is so common in some of the developing countries that some voluntary services overseas offer recruits an injection of gammaglobulin, which protects against it for about six months. A curiosity associated with the illness is that an epidemic may alter the sex ratio of children born to a community after an epidemic, apparently by suppressing male births.

RISKS OF VARIOUS FOODS

To sum up, while we still know very little about the long-term risks of food additives and insecticides, in Britain there are two known and avoidable major risks from food: food poisoning, due particularly to staphylococcal toxin or salmonellae; and brucellosis. Of the various foods, milk, meat, seafood and fruit and vegetables are the most likely to be contaminated.

Milk is an ideal substance for germs to grow in, particularly if it is kept at room temperature. Germs may come from infected animals; the dirty hands of milkers or dirty pails or bottles; coughs and sneezes from the farm workers; and flies. Infections that have been associated with milk and its products (but not yoghurt, in which bacteria are killed by the acid) include streptococcal sore throat and scarlet fever; staphylococcal food poisoning; salmonellosis; tuberculosis; brucellosis; and diphtheria. Pasteurization will kill all of these.

Cream tends to concentrate any bacteria which are present in milk; usually, however, there is little more risk from cream up to the time it is prepared. The increased risk after it has been separated from milk is a feature of its packaging — often done by ladling it out by hand into jars using ordinary jugs under conditions that are far from ideal, such as in a farmhouse kitchen. Cream may or may not be heat-treated before or after this packaging, and if germs are present in the finished product storage at room temperature afterwards allows them to multiply and cause outbreaks of food poisoning.

Meat and poultry are also ideal growth media for germs. They have been linked with outbreaks of staphylococcal and clostridial food poisoning and of salmonellosis. If not thoroughly cooked, meat may contain larvae of worms which can hatch in the digestive system.

Seafood may be contaminated by handling or by sewage containing typhoid or cholera germs or viruses such as that of infectious hepatitis.

Fruit and vegetables are both relatively poor growth media for germs, protazoa or worms, and so tend to be contaminated only on the surface. The organisms, which are killed by cooking, can usually be readily washed off or killed by using a mild disinfectant solution, or raw fruit can be peeled.

Finally, if any carrier of viruses, bacteria, amoebae or worms directly handles prepared food, as in a restaurant, there is a real risk of food poisoning. The risk can be eliminated only by proper supervision of all food-handlers, which includes full medical check-ups if they develop any digestive upset.

Chapter 4

OVER-THE-COUNTER MEDICINES

MEDICINES fall into two main categories: those sold only on a doctor's prescription (the so-called 'ethical preparations'), and those which can be bought over the counter. Even though Britain has a virtually free health service, probably less than a quarter of people with symptoms seek medical advice, and many people (rather more than a third of the total) prefer to treat their own complaints – at least at first. Self-prescribed medicines are big business; they form a third of all drugs taken in Britain, with pain-killers, tonics, skin medicines and laxatives heading the list. These often help the patient, physically and psychologically, and since random surveys have shown that only a third of people think that they have had perfect health in the previous fortnight it is difficult to see how the existing health services would cope if all treatment was prescribed by a doctor.

The chief drawbacks of self-medication are that it may delay the correct treatment of a serious but unrecognized disease or that the medicines themselves may have some harmful effects. The first hazard is more theoretical than real. People who take two or more self-prescribed medicines tend to consult their doctor more than those who take none or only one, and research has shown that people can distinguish between the 'trivial' and the 'serious' illness, treating themselves for one and going to their general practitioner for the other. Furthermore, even after having obtained a first prescription from their doctor many people prefer to buy a repeat supply from the chemist rather than spend time in a crowded waiting room. The government has recognized the large part played by self-prescribing by controlling advertising to ensure that unjustified claims are not made to the public.

Hence the second drawback of self-medication, the harmful effects, is more important. At worst, serious and life-threatening illness may be caused when a drug medically prescribed for one person is given to someone else – 'try these tablets, they worked wonders for me'. Most people recognize the dangers of this action where pills are concerned but seem readier to try a friend's skin ointment, although in practice modern skin preparations contain powerful drugs which may be absorbed into the bloodstream through inflamed skin. To some extent this danger applies to medicines sold over the counter. Drugs that are quite safe for adults may be hazardous to the very young or the very old.

In assessing the dangers of self-medication the harmful effects should be seen in the perspective of the benefit or potential benefit obtained.

ASPIRIN AND OTHER PAIN-KILLERS

Probably half of all medicines sold without prescriptions are pain-killers (analgesics). Most of these contain some form of aspirin, either by itself or mixed with other pain-killers such as codeine. The amount of aspirin consumed is vast: 2,000 tons a year for the population of Britain or two tablets a week for every member of the population, while 2 per cent of men and 9 per cent of women take aspirin every day of their lives. Some take it for headaches, others for some sort of rheumatism – both conditions in which aspirin is often effective – but an appreciable number of people take it for nerves or tiredness, or to induce sleep – all conditions for which aspirin is probably useless. Even so, this high volume of consumption, and the benefits aspirin brings set against the relatively few adverse effects, mean that it is a relatively safe drug – a feature that caused the distinguished Royal physician, Lord Horder, to say that it remained the most valuable weapon in the doctor's armamentarium. Certainly in orthodox medicine it remains the standard treatment for rheumatic fever and most types of arthritis.

In the last twenty years, however, doctors have become aware that aspirin may also do harm. A quarter of people taking it find it causes indigestion, while laboratory tests show that just under three quarters of everybody eating aspirin loses a small amount of blood (about a teaspoonful) in the intestines. In most people such a small loss does little harm, but in 10–15 per cent it may lead to anaemia. This bleeding is due to the irritant effect of aspirin on the stomach lining, which occurs whether tablets are taken before or after meals. With tablets specially prepared so that the aspirin is not released until they have reached the intestine (enteric-coated preparations) this risk is less. A few people may bleed severely after taking aspirin, particularly if it is taken with alcohol, which doubles the risk. Such a serious bleeding episode usually comes out of the blue and is not related to the patient's age, sex or any existing allergy. Aspirin is also thought to be a factor in causing serious bleeding in about half of patients who develop this complication of gastric or duodenal ulceration.

In children aspirin is also a more frequent cause of stomach bleeding than is usually thought. But the main risk to children, particularly toddlers who may mistake attractive preparations of aspirin for sweets, is aspirin poisoning. In adults suicide attempts with aspirin are common (20,000 cases a year, or 10 per cent of the total), and at all ages overdosage may result in serious poisoning – with sickness, overbreathing, headaches, flushing, drowsiness and coma. Poisoning produces complex alterations in the body chemistry, which sometimes need the full resources of a specialist hospital poisons unit to put them right. With lesser amounts, aspirin overdosage may cause deafness, ringing in the ears, dullness in the head and stomach upsets.

A very few people are truly allergic to aspirin and develop severe asthma if they take it. Such people are usually over thirty and may have taken aspirin on many previous occasions without any ill-effects. They usually have no other allergies, but may suffer from polyps in the nose, migraine or sinusitis. Though aspirin sensitivity is rare, it is important because its effects may be grave, even fatal, and the sufferer may well also be sensitive to many other different types of pain-killers. Aspirin also affects the kidney – trivially according to most people, though some think it may occasionally do so seriously. This problem is discussed below, with the effect of other pain-killers on the urinary systems.

Recent research has suggested that aspirin may have other, as yet unproved, effects on the body. Test-tube experiments show that it can affect blood-clotting by an action on the platelets (blood cells which play an important part in triggering clotting) and one of the blood proteins. Such an effect may have advantages and disadvantages. In patients with rheumatoid arthritis who had been treated with aspirin for a long time there was a much lower incidence of clotting diseases compared with other patients (a seventh of the expected number of coronaries and a fifth of the expected number of strokes). On the other hand, there was no difference between the two groups in the incidence of dangerous clotting in the legs after surgical operation. This has led some authorities to suggest that a trial should be set up of the general public taking one aspirin a day to see whether this cuts down the amount of arteriosclerosis and its effects, particularly coronary heart disease. The results of yet more recent surveys have, however, not confirmed such wide differences in the incidence of blood-clotting disorders between those taking aspirin regularly and those not, and the whole question is still unanswered.

The effect on blood-clotting may be dangerous in patients with haemophilia who are given transfusions of blood taken from people who have consumed aspirin – and, since 37 per cent of blood comes from such donors, obviously precautions are needed. Other effects of aspirin have also been reported in pregnancy, in women who took high doses (ten tablets a day for six months). On average their pregnancies lasted a week longer, labour took 70 per cent (five hours) longer, and they lost more blood during childbirth than other women.

Possibly these effects all occur because aspirin counteracts the actions of prostaglandins, substances in the body which among other things may play an important part in the muscular contractions of the uterus during childbirth. Finally, laboratory research has shown that taking aspirin may considerably reduce the amount of vitamin C in the blood platelets, and so feasibly somebody on a poor diet who was taking aspirin regularly might develop scurvy (p. 57).

Codeine is a different type of pain-killer from aspirin but is fairly effective and does not have its serious side-effects. Its chief drawback is that it produces considerable constipation (a property which makes it valuable in treating conditions such as traveller's diarrhoea; p. 127) and for this reason it is usually combined with other pain-killers such as aspirin (compound codeine tablets).

Phenacetin, a moderately good analgesic, is also rarely taken by itself but combined with other pain-killers or even bromide, a largely out-of-date sleeping powder. Excessive use of phenacetin may darken the blood since it alters some of the red pigment inside the red blood cells to a form called methaemoglobin, which is brown. But the most serious effect of phenacetin is on the urinary system, an action recognized only comparatively recently and still the subject of some controversy, though in 1974 the British government restricted its use to doctors' prescriptions only. This aspect is discussed below under 'analgesic nephropathy'.

Because of this effect on the kidney phenacetin has tended to be supplanted by paracetamol, which does not damage the kidneys and which – like codeine and phenacetin – does not produce irritation of or bleeding from the stomach. Its pain-killing effect is something between that of aspirin and compound codeine tablets, but it has one major drawback – that self-poisoning is easy with comparatively small doses and has serious, even lethal, effects. The minimum dose that may cause illness is only between six and twelve times that normally used in treatment and this may seriously damage the liver, heart or blood cells. The most dangerous of these is the effect on the liver, which kills about a quarter of those who develop jaundice – and this may not come on for a day or two after taking the tablet. Every year about 900 people are admitted to hospitals in Britain having taken an overdose of paracetamol tablets, and some thirty-five of them die.

Analgesic nephropathy

Undoubtedly, however, the most serious danger in taking pain-killers is their effect in producing kidney disease. Doctors call this condition 'analgesic nephropathy', but many experts insist that instead it should be called 'phenacetin nephropathy', to indicate what they consider to be the chief or only culprit. There is still a lot of controversy among specialists about this, but the answers are of more than academic importance because they might mean that sales of analgesic other than phenacetin will have to be restricted. For this reason, the phenacetin story is worth telling in some detail.

For some years doctors recognized that some people took phenacetin-containing tablets because they thought these gave them a 'lift', waking them up and helping them work better. Others were addicted to them because of psychological troubles and would go to great lengths to deny that they had taken or were consuming phenacetin and to go on obtaining supplies even though they had been warned against them.

One of the places most intensively studied was Huskvarna, a small town in Sweden which manufactures explosives. During the 1919 influenza pandemic some of the workers were prescribed tablets containing phenacetin and many continued to take these, saying that they improved their work and acted as a stimulant. Tablets became acceptable on social occasions and efforts to persuade the inhabitants to abandon the habit (which included setting up a special clinic) were met with hostility. The incidence of kidney disease in the town rose to a remarkably high level, three times that of another town of the same size in Sweden where tablets were not taken in this way. Thus about two thirds of patients seen in Huskvarna with chronic pyelonephritis (inflammation of the kidney) had a history of abusing analgesics in this way. But, since a law was passed in 1961 restricting the purchase of phenacetin to doctors' prescriptions only, the consumption of phenacetin has fallen to a tenth of what it was, while the incidence of kidney disease has fallen to roughly the same level as for the general population.

There have been many other similar reports of abuse of tablets containing phenacetin, and of phenacetin nephropathy – including accounts from Switzerland, Australia and South Africa – and most have stressed that phenacetin-addiction is a feature of people with inadequate personalities. At one time analgesic abuse was thought to be rare in Britain, but specialists here have now shown that it occurs quite frequently and that the features of the illness are much the same as elsewhere. Thus doctors in Glasgow found that there were five times as many women as men with the condition, that they tended to be middle-aged with psychiatric disorders, and that they often denied taking the tablets – which were rarely taken for 'true' pain but commonly for psychological reasons.

About a third of patients with analgesic nephropathy will deny that they have ever abused pain-killers, and a third will continue to go on abusing them even when the danger has been fully explained. Most patients start by taking the tablets for psychological pain and then find that the codeine and caffeine contained in the compound tablets alter their mood. Abusers come from families with a high prevalence of alcoholism, analgesic abuse and psychiatric disorders, and they may well abuse other drugs as well. Personality tests show that they are passive, introverted and neurotic. Analgesic abuse is also common in patients with psychiatric disorders, being found in over a fifth of patients seen in one Scottish mental hospital, many of whom also had a high incidence of anaemia, kidney failure and previous operations for stomach ulcers.

Research by two London kidney specialists suggested that analgesic kidney disease was far commoner here than generally thought: there might be as many as 500 deaths from this cause each year in England and Wales alone, some unrecognized because the diagnosis was unsuspected. These doctors also emphasized that after a surgical operation (often on the stomach) these patients not uncommonly died. Certainly we know that post-mortem examinations in London teaching hospitals show that between 8 and 15 per cent of patients have analgesic kidney disease, while between 20 and 30 per cent of patients considered for treatment on the artificial kidney machine in Australia have been referred because of it.

The principal argument has centred on whether phenacetin is the sole culprit. Most people with analgesic kidney disease have usually taken tablets containing a mixture of two or three pain-killers, and, though these have almost invariably contained phenacetin, laboratory studies in animals have shown that substances such as aspirin may also affect the kidney. Moreover, patients seen by kidney specialists tend to be highly selected and not representative of the population as a whole. One careful community survey has shown just how many people may be taking pain-killing tablets every day without any ill-effect at all. Of almost 3,000 women living in a Welsh industrial valley, fifty admitted taking over four analgesic tablets a day but even so none of them had evidence of obvious kidney damage.

Quite possibly, therefore, other factors such as climate or urinary infection may determine whether continuous phenacetin taking harms the kidney or not. A long-term prospective trial now being carried out by the World Health Organization should eventually answer this question, but to many doctors outside the argument the message that phenacetin is *the* culprit is now as clear as that cigarette smoking causes lung cancer. Thousands of tons of aspirin have been consumed all over the world for a century, yet the recognition of analgesic kidney disease is comparatively recent. In patients with the disease who stop taking phenacetin but go on taking analgesics the function of the kidney tends to deteriorate much more slowly than those who do not make this change. In countries where over-the-counter sales of phenacetin have been banned or phenacetin has been voluntarily removed the incidence of nephropathy has fallen steeply. Finally, at least six countries now either restrict sales of phenacetin or require boxes of tablets containing it to carry warning labels about the danger to health.

With so much research going on into the effects of phenacetin not surprisingly other effects from the drug have been described, particularly the development of cancers of the urinary system. The hospital serving Huskvarna reported that ten out of fifteen patients with cancer of the main collecting area of the kidney had abused phenacetin – eight of these had analgesic nephropathy as well – and in Sweden as a whole no fewer than sixty-two cases of this type of cancer have been reported in phenacetin abusers. It is not known how many of these people had smoked, another cause of this type of cancer (p. 248), and possibly the two factors could add to one another.

Finally, two other rarer conditions have been described in people who had abused phenacetin: gross narrowing of the middle third of the ureter in three patients – all of whom also had analgesic nephropathy – and dementia in eight patients.

Research subsequent to the latter finding has shown that microscopically the brains of such people may show changes similar to those seen in a rare condition called Alzheimer's disease. As many as a third of patients with analgesic abuse may show abnormalities of the nervous system, or abnormal brain waves, and possibly taking vast quantities of phenacetin may cause advanced changes in the brain as well.

PURGATIVES

Every year the British public spends some £6 million on purgatives (cathartics or laxatives are other generic names). In most cases there is no evidence that these are needed, but people have the mistaken idea that they need a daily bowel motion for health, a concept started by old-fashioned nursery toilet-training and sedulously fostered by many patent medicine manufacturers. In fact, there is a wide variation in bowel habit perfectly compatible with normal health. Purgatives may so completely empty the bowels that they do not fill up again for a few days; since the person cannot open his bowels over this interval he presumes that he is still constipated and increases the dose of the purgative, or switches to a new one.

Apart from this ineffectiveness, purgatives may also do harm. At their simplest, the effects consist of flatulence and vague discomfort in the lower part of the abdomen; at the worst, they may obscure the symptoms of serious illness, or increase the risks of conditions such as acute appendicitis or intestinal obstruction by making the intestines more active and even perforating them. Long-term abuse of purgatives may also severely affect not only the intestines but also other parts of the body. Addiction to purgatives is not uncommon and because patients may deny that they take them at all the diagnosis may be very difficult, and even the prospects of weaning people off them are not very good.

Doctors classify purgatives into three main groups: bulk, such as agar, bran and salts; lubricant, such as liquid (medicinal) paraffin; and irritant, such as senna and cascara. Excessive amounts of agar (a seaweed preparation) and bran may rarely obstruct the intestine and require a surgical operation to relieve them; on the other hand, some experts have argued that some diseases in modern man arise because of too little bulk in his food (p. 50). Salts act rather differently from the other bulk purgatives: they draw fluid out of the wall of the bowel to increase the volume of the contents inside it and so provoke the intestine to contract. This may deplete the body of water and salts, particularly potassium, resulting in kidney damage, weakness of the muscles and loss of weight.

Liquid paraffin may reduce the absorption of fat-soluble vitamins, which is a particularly undesirable effect in pregnancy, when the woman needs more than usual. It also irritates the skin around the anus because it leaks through the final valve of the intestinal passages. Another risk, which is seen particularly in old people who are run down, is that when being swallowed small quantities of the bland paraffin may enter the lungs and cause pneumonia; this also occurs in people who use nose sprays containing paraffin. Does paraffin cause cancer of the bowels? One research project did find that compared with people without cancer twice as many patients with cancer of the digestive tract had used medicinal paraffin – but any risk was discounted because it seemed likely that paraffin might have been taken to treat conditions tending to give rise to cancer rather than to have caused cancer itself.

The irritant purgatives may produce severe purging with a condition similar to that seen with salts if they are used for a prolonged period. In particular, loss of the element potassium from the body may cause muscle weakness, disturbances of the heart rhythm and kidney disorder. In addition, they may cause considerable enlargement of the colon, probably by destroying its nerve supply. Phenolphthalein may produce an irritating rash as well as colouring the urine pink. Finally, a substance called oxyphenisatin has now been withdrawn from sale in Britain, though it is still available in Australia and the USA. This has been recognized as a cause of fatigue and discomfort in the abdomen as well as a serious type of jaundice.

DIGESTIVE REMEDIES

Some half of indigestion remedies are bought over the counter, and (apart from mild constipation or diarrhoea) these normally do little harm unless excessive amounts are taken. In patients with heart disease the sodium absorbed from normal quantities of baking soda (sodium bicarbonate), a commonly used remedy, may cause heart failure while, in patients already being treated with tetracycline antibiotics, aluminium hydroxide may combine with these and prevent their being absorbed from the intestines. But in general, as with other self-prescribed remedies, the real dangers come from their gross and prolonged over-use. As with other remedies, people with inadequate personalities may become addicted to indigestion remedies and persist in taking them even when advised to stop. The main danger with alkali indigestion mixtures, such as sodium bicarbonate, is that the body's chemistry becomes alkaline and that the level of calcium in the bloodstream rises (similar to that seen in people taking excessive quantities of vitamin D; p. 58). Both these tendencies are made worse by the large quantities of milk which people with indigestion often drink as well. Eventually the calcium level in the bloodstream may fall, giving rise to irritability of the muscles. Calcium also becomes deposited in the kidney, and serious or fatal kidney disease may develop.

Another risk of a frequently taken substance has been recognized only fairly recently: a nervous disease linked with taking clioquinol, a chemical mildly active against some bowel parasites such as *Giardia lamblia* and amoeba (p. 77) and contained in preparations such as Enterovioform. This was introduced for preventing traveller's diarrhoea in the 1930s, and at one time was thought to be entirely safe – even for prolonged use. In the late 1950s, however, doctors in Japan described an outbreak of a peculiar illness called subacute myelo-optic neuropathy, or SMON. This usually started with diarrhoea and intense pain in the abdomen, and was followed by pains, tingling and numbness in the legs and a staggering gait. Half the patients developed weakness of their muscles and a quarter impaired vision. Though the main features of the illness tended to disappear (only 11 per cent of patients got worse or died), most patients were left with persistent pain and numbness in their legs. Altogether between 10,000 and 12,000 people developed this illness.

At first the Japanese doctors suspected that a virus infection was responsible. But later they came to believe that the illness was due to clioquinol. Research showed that no case of SMON developed in patients with a digestive upset who had not taken clioquinol, but that the incidence was about 17 per cent in those who did. All this led to the substance being banned by the Japanese Health Ministry in 1970; the following year only ten cases were reported in the whole country.

The arguments about the role of clioquinol are still continuing. Some experts maintain that the Japanese have a racial susceptibility to it, a feature which is certainly recognized for other drugs. Others point out that in this outbreak large doses of clioquinol powder (rather than tablets) had been taken over long periods. Even so, a few cases have now been reported from Australia and the Netherlands, as well as one in Britain, while previous reports of occasional difficulties with vision or nervous disturbances in German or American patients who were taking clioquinol have now been unearthed.

At present there seems to be little danger from taking normal amounts of clioquinol for a short period, say, over the average holiday. The risks of developing SMON for a Londoner taking it for six weeks or more have been estimated as one in ten, with a good chance of complete recovery in a few days if clioquinol is stopped straight away. Even so, the obvious question doctors will ask is 'how much preventive value does clioquinol have anyway?', an aspect discussed further on p. 128.

OTHER MEDICINES

Many other medicines may do harm, though much less frequently than those discussed already. If they are drunk, some skin preparations – particularly linaments containing camphor, aconite and oil of wintergreen – may cause serious poisoning. Excessive doses of vitamins may be harmful (p. 55) and cough mixtures may cause vomiting. Phenylpropanolamine, a substance which decongests the nose and which is present in many 'cold-cures', often raises the blood pressure slightly in normal people, but in patients being treated for high blood pressure it may totally reverse the beneficial effects of drug treatment. In patients with depression who are treated with monoamine oxidase inhibitor drugs phenylpropanolamine may raise the blood pressure so dangerously that brain haemorrhage results, an effect also seen if these patients take cheese or Marmite.

Finally, doctors have recently warned that there is a risk of serious addiction to yet other preparations sold over the counter, such as Dr Collis Browne's chlorodyne. These contain morphine, and addiction to these preparations can reach a stage where an individual drinks thirty bottles a day. The Department of Health has required the makers of Dr Collis Browne's Compound to reduce its morphine content, but this and other morphine-containing medicines can still be bought over the counter.

Chapter 5

EXERCISE AND SPORT

FRESH air and exercise, the Victorian prescription for everything from constipation to homosexuality, are still seen as necessarily healthy by most people. Current medical concern with the dangers of a sedentary life has led to enthusiastic claims for the value of home gymnasia and bouts of violent activity on squash courts. Jogging has not caught on in Britain as it has in the USA, but many middle-aged men are beginning to look around for an easy way of keeping fit, or at least postponing their heart attack for a few years (p. 300). Unfortunately, exercise does have its hazards; and to appreciate these some understanding is needed of the way that muscles work. In exercising muscles the blood flow may be thirty times faster than at rest, the amount of oxygen used 100 times the resting value and the rise in temperature may be up to 2–3°C. This great increase in muscular activity means that much more blood is pumped back to the heart, aided by quicker and deeper breathing, while blood is switched from relatively inessential parts, such as the intestines, to the general circulation. Blood flow to the skin may be increased as much as four times, as both sweating and the generalized widening of the small blood-vessels in the skin help to get rid of the heat generated by exercise and so keep the body temperature down.

Training increases muscle bulk and strength by increasing the size of the individual muscle fibres and diminishing the amount of fat between them. The bones and ligaments also become stronger, and more air can be drawn into the lungs. Some of the most definite effects are seen on the heart. This increases up to 15 per cent in size, particularly in endurance athletes, and tends to beat more slowly; a resting pulse of 40–60 beats a minute compared with one in an untrained person of 70–80 is not unusual. But the athlete's heart also pumps out more blood with every stroke – in other words, it can put out more blood at a slower rate. During exercise the heart rate speeds up less in the trained than in the untrained, but the amount of blood pumped out may be half as much again: 30–36 litres a minute in an athlete, compared with 24 litres a minute in a sedentary person. The athlete's body can also extract more oxygen from the bloodstream. The changes in fatty acid levels in the bloodstream between sedentary people and athletes are particularly pronounced. Even at rest the levels are significantly lower in athletes, they do not increase with age as they do in the untrained, and the rise occurring during exercise is much less. All this suggests, among other things, that training enables people to burn up fats much more efficiently, even when they are not taking exercise. Exercise also affects the so-called fibrinolytic system in the blood, which is a continuous process normally dissolving any small particles of blood-clots in the blood-vessels, formed to repair small areas of damage or injury. After exercise fibrinolysis is increased – in other words, the blood can deal more readily with any clots present in the vessels.

EXERCISE AND CORONARY HEART DISEASE

There are two types of exercise. Isometric or static exercises involve muscle contraction without movement, as when the fingers of the two hands are linked and the arm muscles tensed in the action of pulling the hands apart. This type of exercise is much used in body-building courses but has little effect on the pulse, respiration or indeed physical fitness. Rhythmic or dynamic exercise includes gymnastics and most outdoor sports and may protect against illness, though until recently the evidence that it did so was only circumstantial. The most important illness that is influenced by exercise is coronary heart disease (CHD), which includes angina pectoris (a cramping pain in the chest arising in the heart muscle) and myocardial infarction (the classic coronary attack). Death from CHD seems to be comparatively rare in primitive communities, even after allowing for the obvious difficulties in collecting reliable data.

Statisticians have shown that the death rate from CHD increases step by step with the number of motorcars in a community. Also as industry has become more and more mechanized the number of really heavy jobs has declined, corresponding with the so-called epidemic of CHD in the developed countries. But which of the known possible coronary risk factors absent in primitive or non-mechanized societies plays the most important part: heredity, diet, smoking, stress or physical activity?

So far as exercise is concerned we have been helped by some research done on comparable groups in civilized communities. The classical work was done by Professor J. N. Morris and his colleagues of the Medical Research Council's Social Medicine Research Unit, who compared the incidence of CHD in a large group of bus drivers with that in bus conductors. Both groups lived under much the same social circumstances and were served by the same health and welfare services, so that the observations are likely to have been reliable. But the drivers' job was strictly sedentary, whereas the conductors were estimated to climb the height of the Empire State Building every day. Statistics adjusted for age showed that every year 2·7 out of every 1,000 drivers developed CHD, compared with only 1·9 of the conductors. What was more, coronaries occurred at a younger age and were more fatal in the drivers than in the conductors, the death rates in the first three months being 47 per cent and 29 per cent respectively. On the other hand, compared with the drivers, conductors had double the amount of angina.

Morris and his team suggested three main possible explanations for these findings. The first possibility was physique and constitution as well as self-selection for the job. Obviously such factors have to be considered, since, for example, one would have to be keen on heavy exercise in the open air (as well as able to do it) to be a Canadian lumberjack. Certainly Morris found that the size of their first uniforms showed that his London bus drivers had been fatter than conductors right at the start of their jobs. The second factor was some kind of mental strain involved in driving buses. This again might have partly explained the difference between drivers and conductors, except he then found that drivers of London underground trains (presumably exposed to less or different types of strain) had much the same pattern of CHD as the bus drivers.

The third possibility was that exercise reduced the incidence of CHD. This was the easiest one to study because the incidence of CHD could be determined in other groups who were identical except for the amount of exercise they took at work. Morris found that there was a similar gradient among postal workers – sedentary groups (such as telephonists, clerks and executives) having a higher total incidence and death rate from coronaries, but a lower incidence of angina, compared with the postmen – who took active exercise at work.

The research then turned to a large-scale analysis of death rates from CHD according to occupation. Morris and his team found that there was a distinct dividing line between heavy and light work, people being twice as likely to die in the latter. But this difference was not related to social class because the death rate in women from CHD was found to bear no relation to whether their husband's work was heavy or light.

This thesis has been independently confirmed by research on otherwise comparable groups carrying out strenuous and sedentary activities, such as forestry workers and civil servants. In American railwaymen the annual death rate from CHD was 7·6 for labourers, 10·6 for signalmen and 11·8 for clerks. The fact that an active job may lower the risk of dying after a coronary was supported by a British Medical Research Council project, which found that the death rate in coronary patients treated in hospital in the first month was

8·2 per cent for heavy workers, 13·8 per cent for active workers and 18·8 per cent for light workers.

Given all the ifs and buts, which research workers in this field always stress, there seems little doubt that the amount of CHD in people doing the same work is directly related to how much or what kind of exercise they take during their leisure. Possibly even walking to work gives some protection, although a more recent study by Morris emphasizes that much heavier exercise is needed. In 1968–70 his group asked almost 17,000 male sedentary civil servants to fill in a questionnaire describing all their daily activities, social circumstances, and medical and personal behaviour. This survey included an account of the exercise the men took apart from their work, on two days, a Friday (normally working) and Saturday (free). Since then the group has obtained any sickness and death certificates for these men, so that they could find out which of them had developed CHD.

By the end of September 1972, 232 men had had an episode of CHD. For each of them the computer chose two control men who had not had such an attack, and the three records were then examined without knowing which were the patients and which the controls to see whether there were any links with exercise. The findings confirmed what the early results had suggested: that people taking vigorous exercise were significantly less likely to have CHD. Only twenty-three of the men known to have had a coronary had taken vigorous exercise, compared with an expected number of 55·5. Among the men not doing vigorous exercise, 191 of them had had coronaries, compared with an expected number of 158·5.

By vigorous high-intensity activity Morris and his team meant two things: firstly, recreation, sports and games requiring peaks of energy output of 7·5 kilocalories (kcal.) per minute or more (this is the same level as 'heavy' industrial work); and, secondly, that this should go on uninterrupted for more than thirty minutes. The activities which produced this level of energy output included: swimming, tennis, sailing as crew, hill-climbing and dancing; morning exercises; heavy gardening and do-it-yourself, such as clearing scrub or concreting; major car maintenance; brisk walking in town, or over rough country; running; cycling; and climbing over 500 stairs daily (to the top of St Paul's). The greater the amount of vigorous exercise that was taken, the less the risk of CHD. But other less heavy types of work, such as lawn-mowing, playing golf and strolling to work did not seem to be linked with protection against CHD. Interestingly enough, vigorous exercise appeared partially to protect against the known increased risk of CHD in cigarette smokers (p. 244). In men taking vigorous exercise the relative risks were 36 per cent of the average for non-smokers and 50 per cent for smokers; in those not taking vigorous exercise they were 75 per cent and 185 per cent respectively. In other words, on these results, *strictly for lessening the risk of coronary disease*, it would seem to be better to take vigorous exercise and to smoke cigarettes rather than do neither.

Obviously these results raise almost as many questions as they answer – in particular, how long the group of men studied had been taking vigorous exercise and why. They seemed unlikely to be particularly health-conscious since as many people taking vigorous exercise smoked cigarettes as those who did not. Also, since the population studied was restricted to a middle-class, white-collar, stable group, it seems important to study this problem in other groups, and then, as Morris suggests, to try persuading inactive men to start a programme of increasingly vigorous exercise.

If the conclusions drawn from these results are correct, how does exercise lessen the risk of CHD? Virtually every adult in a developed country has atherosclerosis – deposits of fatty material (atheroma) in the lining of the major arteries in the body (p. 44), together with the reaction of the surrounding tissues – and it is not uncommon to find after death old clots in some of the small arteries supplying the heart muscle. But only when these deposits excessively narrow the main blood-vessels or a clot forms on a deposit blocking the vessel do symptoms result. Narrowing of the coronary arteries may cause angina if the heart muscle cannot be supplied with enough oxygen during exercise, while a blood clot (or thrombosis) may block the blood-supply to some of the heart muscle, destroying it (myocardial infarction). Research in people taking vigorous exercise has shown that they have less thrombosis in the small blood-vessels in the heart, but just as much atherosclerosis as in the hearts of sedentary people. So atherosclerosis does not seem to go hand in hand with thrombosis. Interestingly enough the independence of these two conditions has been confirmed by examining carefully kept pathology records for the past seventy years, which has shown that on average the amount of coronary atherosclerosis has changed very little, though coronary thrombosis has swelled into an epidemic.

Another important difference between the hearts of sedentary and active people is that the smaller arteries inside the heart muscle are usually wider in the latter. So it may be that vigorous exercise enlarges the arteries supplying the heart muscle, and also trains the heart to cope better with sudden stress. Morris's research suggests that it is not the total number of calories one burns up but how quickly that is important; the exercise must be vigorous enough to produce and maintain a 'training' effect on the circulation. Other possible factors are the lower level of fatty acids and the increased fibrinolysis in the bloodstream which occur in those taking regular exercise. Certainly, if exercise is proved to benefit the heart, it will be important to know how little is enough, for many sedentary people would like to take exercise but have difficulty in doing so or in finding the time. Thus recent research at Oxford suggests that as little as seventeen to twenty minutes' vigorous exercise three times a week significantly improves athletic performance, reduces overweight, increase muscle tone and produces a lower resting pulse rate. Possibly this might have an effect on the development of CHD. A book by two Scots physiologists, J. V. G. A. Durnin and R. Passmore, *Energy, Work and*

Leisure – which is engagingly witty and a mine of detailed information on energy expenditure – comments: 'We would like to see a law enacted compelling those who build large blocks of offices to install squash courts and a swimming bath in the basement. This would be a sensible public health measure.'

Another way of solving the problem of exercise for the sedentary would be official encouragement of bicycles for transport in our cities, solving several problems at the same time. Vigorous recreational cycling involves energy expenditure of a least 7·5 kcal. per minute – Morris's figure for protection against CHD. Anybody who has tried to cycle into a big city, however, knows how unpleasant – and dangerous – an experience it usually is; perhaps some difficulties could be solved by making bus/cycle-only lanes the rule in all our major streets, and enforcing this use.

Finally there is the psychological benefit of taking exercise – not only experienced subjectively as an increased feeling of fitness, but also detectable objectively as an increase in visual speed tests and ability to concentrate. At present these psychological benefits seem to be the main reason for using programmes of gradually increasing exercise in treating patients with known CHD, either angina or previous myocardial infarction. Several of these projects have been initiated at various centres. To start with, patients exercise to increase their mobility, and then to increase the strength of various muscle groups; this is followed by daily walks which increase in length and pace. Finally, a strong endurance component is added – jogging, running on the spot and swimming. A high level of activity can then be maintained by introducing competition; often the social aspects of this later part of the programme keep up the participants' enthusiasm. The early part of the programme is often supervised by a doctor, but this is more to reassure the patients than for medical reasons, as fresh episodes of CHD during exercise seem to be very rare. So far there have been no statistically controlled studies of the value of exercise in preventing a recurrence of illness in patients with known CHD, but enough doctors, and patients, seem to be convinced of its value for new programmes to be starting all the time.

EFFECTS OF TOTAL INACTIVITY

No one knows just how long somebody has to lead a sedentary life before he runs an increased risk of a coronary attack. But for somebody who is completely inactive certain short-term effects are seen within a few weeks. In ill patients the dangers of prolonged rest in bed are well known, and were summed up by Richard Asher in a passage of Churchillian rotundity:

Look at a patient lying in bed. What a pathetic picture he makes! The blood clotting in his veins, the lime draining from his bones, the scybala stacking up in his colon, the flesh rotting from his seat, the urine leaking from his distended bladder, and the spirit evaporating from his soul.

In completely normal people, on the other hand, the effects of prolonged rest in bed are much less serious than Asher rightly describes for ill patients. There is no evidence that prolonged inactivity harms the heart, lungs or digestive system. Even so, everybody has experienced the shaky, dizzy feeling which occurs on first getting up after being in bed some time. This is due partly to a loss of the sense of balance and partly to a failure of the blood-vessels to make the usual adjustments to standing upright. Why such adjustments should fail nobody knows.

There are three more serious changes in body metabolism which affect the normal person or the ill patient lying in bed. Firstly, some of the muscle substance is broken down, so that by the end of the second week the body is losing more nitrogen than it is taking in. This process affects particularly the antigravity muscles of the limbs – those associated with posture and walking – and is equivalent to a loss of 1·7 kg. of muscle after six weeks of bed rest. Once the person gets up and is normally active again, muscle strength is restored in about four weeks.

The second serious change is a loss of calcium from the bones, which begins at the end of the first week and leads to the bones becoming thinner than normal. Some 23 gm. of calcium are lost during six weeks' bed rest, and its increased concentration in the urine leads to the third hazard – an increased risk of stones forming in the kidney. During rest in bed the prolonged dependent position of the kidneys means that stagnant pools of urine collect at the bases of the kidneys, and the raised level of calcium in these pools may precipitate out as salts and lead to the formation of stones.

Other complications of bed rest which are often mentioned – such as constipation and difficulty in passing urine – seem to be due to the psychological pressures of the average hospital ward. Again, another frequent and dreaded complication – the formation of blood clots in the deep veins of the legs which pass to the lungs, sometimes with fatal results – does not apparently occur in really healthy people, however long they stay in bed. This is because several other factors are needed to cause clotting, or thrombosis, in the deep veins of the leg: damage to the veins, slowing of the flow of blood and an increased tendency of the blood to clot. Some or all of these factors are present in patients during and after a surgical operation, and deep-vein thrombosis occurs in some 30 per cent of them. Even apparently healthy people may have one abnormality, such as varicose veins, which may lead to clotting under some circumstances. This was seen, for example, during the Second World War in women who slept all night in deck-chairs in air-raid shelters; presumably the position of the legs led to kinking of the veins, which were probably varicose with a sluggish blood flow, and they woke in the morning with a painful thrombosis. Today this complication is seen occasionally in aircraft passengers on a long flight who do not move about as much as they should.

EXERCISE AND EARLY DEATH

If there is still some controversy about the long-term benefit from exercise, most experts now agree that strenuous exercise rarely kills. Death during exercise is almost always due to an undiagnosed complaint, such as a weakness of a small blood-vessel in the brain, present since birth, which bursts during exercise owing to the rise in blood-pressure. Another cause is a rare, hidden infection of the heart muscle itself, called myocarditis, and usually due to a virus.

What effect does exercise have on longevity? Only recently have doctors agreed that it certainly does not shorten life, although it may not prolong it all that much. At one time, having interpreted the usual enlargement of the heart in trained athletes as due to disease, people talked about athlete's or oarsman's heart. Understandably, the distinction between training effect and disease was particularly difficult to draw in rowers since they may have very slow pulse rates and heart murmurs, both of which also occur in heart disease. Another factor contributing to this legend seems to have been the death in 1897 of three well-known British oarsmen, all in their twenties. This led to articles in the medical and lay press about the dangers of rowing, until one oarsman who had known all three of the men revealed that one had died from a ruptured appendix, the second from tuberculosis and the third from an overwhelming infection. Even though the concept of oarsman's heart has been a long time dying, several research projects have confirmed the conclusion that rowing neither lengthens nor shortens life – while the appearance at the Henley Royal Regatta in 1964 of exactly the same Harvard Junior Varsity Crew (including a US senator as bow and captain and an emeritus professor of surgery at stroke) that had won the Grand Challenge Cup fifty years earlier must surely have buried for good any association of a shortened life-span with rowing.

Anecdotal evidence of longevity has also recently been provided for two other sports. A report from Finland has shown that cross-country champion skiers live six to seven years longer than the average man in the population, while the American Medical Joggers Association has stated that there has never been a death from coronary heart disease in a former marathon runner. The results of the post-mortem examination of a famous American marathon runner, who had died of cancer at the age of seventy, are also relevant. This man's athletic career had lasted for almost fifty years and he had run in over 1,000 long-distance races (100 of twenty-five miles or more), the last at the age of sixty-nine. His heart weighed in the upper normal range; the coronary arteries showed some atheroma, but particularly striking was their diameter – which was two or three times greater than normal.

One of the difficulties in arriving at a true assessment of the effect of top-class competitive sport on longevity has always been to collect sufficient details about enough athletes and the causes of their deaths, and then to compare them with a group of similar social class. The importance of this was shown in a study by Sir Alan Rook, then Senior Health Officer at Cambridge University. He found that the expectation of life in a group of students who had entered, or 'matriculated' at, the university between 1860 and 1900 had not changed at all over the years, compared with the general population – in which the expectation is known to have considerably improved – thus confirming statistically the obvious fact that students, then and now, are a highly privileged class. In his research Rook got over this drawback by comparing the university athletes with other student contemporaries. He obtained details of a total of 1,476 Cambridge men from *Alumni Cantabrigienses* (which records all men matriculating at the university) and from death certificates. This total included three groups, as follows. Firstly, 834 sportsmen who had represented the university in four major sports (rowing, cricket, athletics and rugby football – to give the historical order in which these events were recognized by the award of a blue). The second group comprised 382 'intellectuals', defined as those occupying the first four places in the mathematical and classical tripos examinations; these included six men with blues or half-blues (one man obtained a first in classics and blues for both rowing and athletics). The third group were 336 former students chosen at random to fulfil the requirements of the study.

Comparing the various groups, Rook found that on average the intellectuals seemed to live two years longer than the random group and one and a half years longer than the sportsmen. Up to the age of forty, however, the sportsmen seemed to have the best prospects for survival. Life-table calculations showed that the chances of living up to ninety were apparently best for the cricketers, followed by oarsmen, rugby footballers and athletes, in that order. Heavyweight men (rugby backs, oarsmen over 168 lb. and hammer-and-weight men) seemed to have an advantage for survival over the lightweight men until middle age, after which the reverse was true. Finally, the sportsmen seemed twice as likely as the intellectuals, and a third as likely again as the random group, to succumb to accidents and war deaths; violent deaths in the intellectual group were due mainly to mountain accidents.

More recent research by Dr Peter Schnohr of Copenhagen has again eliminated any statistical bias due to social class, since he studied a group of athletes many of whom had not been to university and whose social distribution resembled that of the population as a whole. This project concerned the longevity and causes of death in 307 male athletes, all of them Danish champions, and several with Olympic, world or European honours. The period studied covered 1880 to 1910 and a wide variety of sporting events was included. Schnohr found that between the ages of twenty-five and fifty the mortality was 39 per cent less among the athletes than among men of the same age in the general population, but that after this age the death rates were the same. Whether in fact all these findings merely prove that athletes are a self-selected fit group who have natural advantages over their fellows – at least up to middle age – is not yet known, but the results do prove that participation in top-class sport certainly does not shorten life.

MAJOR DANGERS OF VARIOUS SPORTS

Obviously some sports are more dangerous than others, both in the frequency and in the severity of their inherent risks. It is difficult to compile a 'league table', but some figures provided by Professor Roy Shephard and colleagues at Toronto University are a useful guide. They found that the time a person had to participate before being injured severely enough to take him to a doctor varied greatly according to the sport, from about fifty days for wrestling and football to over twenty years for rowing. Surprisingly, the figure for hockey was the high one of 253 days – and, even more surprisingly, that for boxing the higher one of 275 days.

Boxing

Perhaps the latter finding reflects the fact that at least one of the serious hazards of boxing is now recognized to occur some years after the sport has been given up. Deaths from bleeding into the brain caused by blows received during a professional fight may make newspaper headlines, but they are fortunately comparatively rare – six in Britain since the end of the Second World War. But punch-drunkenness, a condition coming on after some years of boxing, is a much commoner condition, affecting up to 17 per cent of some groups of boxers studied.

Punch-drunkenness is a state of loss of the sense of balance, slurred speech and mental impairment, which may become progressively worse even though the boxer has retired from the ring. It is much commoner in professionals than amateurs, particularly in ones who are not in the top flight but have spent some time as sparring partners to champions or at exhibitions in fairgrounds. Although the condition has now been recognized for well over forty years, up to a few years ago we had little idea of its true prevalence. But the main features were described in a special report by the Royal College of Physicians of London in 1969, and they were amplified in a book, *Brain Damage in Boxers*, by Dr A. H. Roberts, who undertook most of the research. The RCP Committee on Boxing studied a random sample of 250 boxers, or 1·5 per cent of the total number of boxers registered with the British Board of Boxing Control between 1929 and 1955. Every one of these was traced and the available 224 questioned and examined for disease of the nervous system and psychological abnormalities. The wives of the boxers were also seen, and the boxers themselves were asked for their own views on punch-drunkenness. Finally the details of the boxers' professional careers were obtained and checked with contemporary boxing journals and annuals.

No fewer than thirty-seven of the total of 224 boxers studied showed some brain damage, which was disabling in thirteen; on the other hand, probably only one third of these showed features obvious enough for a layman to diagnose punch-drunkenness. Two ex-boxers had such impairment of intellectual function that they were being cared for in a mental hospital, and another fourteen showed some degree of impairment and personality change. The longer the boxing careers, the higher the prevalence of brain damage was found: in boxers aged fifty or over who had boxed for ten years or more almost half had some degree of punch-drunkenness; the proportions for those boxing for six to nine years and five years or less were 17 per cent and 13 per cent respectively. If these conclusions are applied to the whole of Britain, there must be about 200 severely punch-drunk ex-boxers and another 400–500 men with damage detectable only on specialist medical examination. There was also some evidence that the heavier the boxing class, the commoner the occurrence of punch-drunkenness. But Dr Roberts also stressed that during his interviews he often formed the impression that many of the boxers were conscientious, responsible and stable men who had improved their job status. The majority were not socially aggressive, whatever their behaviour had been in the ring.

Other conditions seen on medical examination were weakness of one of the eye muscles in five cases and detachment of the retina with virtual blindness in the eye in two. Both of these conditions were probably due to damage to the eyes received during fights. This is less than the incidence of eye complications previously reported in boxing, and the men can probably recover from them once they stop boxing. Twenty-six boxers were deaf, and in ten of them there was a clear history of ear injury with bleeding from the outer ear canal.

The boxers' own views of the effects of boxing are of some interest, although they were obtained from only three quarters of the group – including only half of those with punch-drunkenness. Of the 165 ex-boxers questioned, four said that they had never seen anybody come to any harm from boxing. Many of the remainder described a condition they had seen, called 'punchy', 'puddled' or 'punch-drunk', with unsteady walking, slurred speech, trembling of the limbs and other features. Some said that they had seen half a dozen such cases – others dozens or fifty – but it was generally agreed that far fewer had been seen since the war, though the men had no hesitation in attributing the condition to boxing and the result of too much punishment.

Some research by Dr J. Johnson in the Manchester area has shown just how serious the mental changes may be in some cases. All but one of his sixteen professional ex-boxers had been lightweights and each had had an average of 200–300 fights, mostly in fairgrounds. The psychiatric disorders were of two main types; forgetfulness, dementia and impotence, often associated with morbid jealousy; and aggressive or paranoid disturbances, often occurring after drinking alcohol, to which the men became increasingly susceptible.

The actual changes in the brain which may be responsible for punch-drunkenness have recently been described from Runwell Hospital in Essex. A medical team there studied the brains of fifteen ex-boxers (two world champions, six national or regional champions and three amateurs). Over half had taken part in more than 300 contests or had had careers lasting fifteen years or more, or both; twelve of the fifteen had shown physical and psychological deterioration before they died. The brain showed four abnormal features: an abnormality of a particular membrane deep in the substance of the brain; scarring in the cerebellum (part of the brain concerned with balance); degeneration of the substantia nigra (responsible for coordination of movements, including speech); and tangles of nerve fibres in the substance of the main part of the brain. Any of these changes might have been due to causes other than boxing but the occurrence of all four together could not be accounted for in this way. Moreover, these changes might explain many of the features of punch-drunkeness, including loss of memory, dementia, loss of balance, and rage reactions.

All the reports about the effects of boxing are careful to point out that our present-day knowledge relates to the times when boxing was much less stringently controlled than today – and that no conclusions can be drawn about the risk of brain damage in professional boxing today. In particular, the risks of amateur boxing seem to be relatively few. Thus a survey of amateur boxing in the Royal Air Force between 1953 and 1966 showed a total of 240 injuries (139 to the head and neck, thirty-nine of the arms and shoulders, and fifty-nine other), though two deaths occurred from head injuries and one man had to be invalided out of the service. Since the RAF began very strict medical control of boxing in 1959 there have been no deaths and statistics for 1960–66 showed that the injury rate was 6·2 per 1,000 'man-bouts' (3·9 of these were injuries of the head and neck). But certainly the need to supervise boxing and boxers **carefully does emerge from the Runwell report:**

A single punch, or even many punches, to the head need not visibly alter the structure of the brain but there is still the danger that, at an unpredictable moment, and for an unknown reason, one or more blows will leave their mark. The destruction of cerebral [brain] tissue will then have begun and, although this will usually be slight enough in the early stages to be undetectable, it may build up, if the boxing continues, until it becomes clinically evident. At this point, however, it could already be too late, for destroyed cerebral tissue can never be replaced, while the further danger exists that the process of degeneration could smoulder on even after the boxing has stopped. It is not suggested that this is a common sequence of events, but that it has occurred occasionally can scarcely be denied.

Evidence to support this cautious view has come recently from a study reported in the *Lancet* of the effects of concussion on brain function. Two New Zealand doctors investigated the recovery rates of young adults admitted to hospital as a result of injuries from sports and traffic accidents. Some had had previous head injuries and some had not. Though there was no difference in the severity of their injuries, the patients who had had concussion before were slower to recover than those admitted with their first head injury. The New Zealand doctors concluded that any episode of concussion destroys some brain cells permanently. Since, however, the brain has plenty of reserve capacity this damage is generally noticeable only in unusual circumstances such as the recovery period after a subsequent injury. Nevertheless each knockout must have an effect – and one which is cumulative.

Soccer, rugby and champion athletics

About a quarter of all football injuries involve the knee or ankle joints, which may be affected by synovitis (inflammation of the joint lining) or by damage to the ligaments surrounding and protecting the joint. Occasionally one of the shock-absorbing cartilages inside the knee joint may become torn and cause it to lock. A further half of the injuries affect muscles, either by direct injury from a blow or indirectly when the muscle fibres are torn by vigorous contraction.

A recently described curiosity in footballers is the occurrence of migraine provoked by heading the ball and characterized by blurred vision, difficulty in speaking and numbness. Heading the ball also probably causes damage to the joints in the neck in professional footballers, and similar damage may occur in other joints as a result of repeated minor injuries.

In rugby football the injuries are traditionally more dramatic, an impression confirmed by some figures for one region produced by an Irish doctor with some twenty years experience of the game. Over this period there were four deaths, three from fracture-dislocations of the bones of the neck and one from an undiagnosed rupture of the spleen. The injuries included 129 to the head, 110 to the shoulder, seventy-seven to other parts of the arm, seventy-five to the knees, forty-two to the ankles, thirty-five to the spine and pelvis and fifty-three leg fractures.

An example of the over-use of muscle is seen in champion swimmers, who may strain their shoulder muscles in training doing up to 50,000 strokes a week. Well-known muscle tears are associated with particular sports and have acquired familiar names such as tennis elbow and leg, golfer's elbow and skier's thumb. In the commonest of these, tennis elbow, the muscle on the outside of the arm just below the elbow joint is slightly torn, and if not properly rested there may be a long period when it is painful to move the wrist backwards, as in playing a backhand drive.

Overtraining in athletes may affect the tendons as well as the muscles and cause severe soreness of the shins – 'shin splints' as it is called in the USA. The cartilage lining the back of the kneecap may become roughened and cause pain, particularly severe on descending stairs; this particularly affects long-distance runners, bicycle-riders and cricketers. Small fractures of bones (stress fractures) may occur in the feet of any athlete, particularly early in the season. All these conditions and the effect they may have on the success of a football team possibly worth several million pounds are reflected in the care leading clubs take to retain their own medical staff, physiotherapists and masseurs ready to start intensive treatment as soon as possible after any injury.

Walking and climbing

Despite the wide publicity given to rescue operations in mountainous areas, every year parties of walkers go off into hilly country hopelessly ill-equipped for any emergency. Even in summer apparently harmless, rounded hills may in fact be a death trap.

The main hazard is hypothermia – loss of body heat leading to a state of mental and physical collapse. The human body functions efficiently only at its normal temperature of 98·4°F. or 37°C. Even a drop of 2°F. in this temperature causes appreciable impairment of mental efficiency, and in normal conditions the internal thermostat prevents any such variation in body heat. Heat is produced by muscular activity, and to a lesser extent by the processes of digestion and chemical breakdown of food. This heat is normally dissipated through the skin, and the rate of heat loss is determined by the rate of blood flow through the skin. If much heat has to be lost, the blood flow is increased and the skin becomes flushed and warm: conversely if heat has to be conserved the skin becomes pale and cold.

The body has limited stores of fuel to maintain its heat production. Walking in hilly country is one of the most demanding forms of physical activity in terms of energy required, and an adult on a walking expedition probably needs at least 4,000 calories a day. If weather conditions are such that heat loss from the body is increased the energy balance may easily become negative and it may become impossible to maintain body heat. This is most likely to occur when wet, cold conditions are combined with high winds. If clothing is not really wind- and waterproof these conditions may cause rapid cooling of the skin, and severe symptoms of exposure may develop within a few hours.

Advice on walking in mountainous areas has been published in booklet form by the British Mountaineering Council. This stresses that it is the combination of fatigue with cold which is especially dangerous, and points out that whole parties have died because they tried to keep moving at all costs rather than resting in some shelter before becoming exhausted.

The symptoms of exposure include unreasonable behaviour, often accompanied by complaints of tiredness and coldness; physical and mental lethargy; slurring of speech; shivering fits; and clumsiness. Once such symptoms develop treatment is a matter of urgency, and this should be aimed at preventing further loss of heat and replacing energy stores. In practice this means extra clothing, shelter from the weather, and hot food and drink.

Clearly, however, prevention is the best policy. Anyone intending to spend a day in hilly country should be aware that mist, gales, heavy rain or even blizzards may descend very quickly. No matter how attractive the weather appears each member of the party should at least have a waterproof jacket or anorak, long trousers and proper footwear. Emergency rations should be carried in addition to any picnic or packed lunch. The emergency ration recommended by the Mountaineering Council, sufficient for six people for twenty-four hours in good conditions, four people in bad, consists of: 6 oz. sugar, one bar of mint cake, one pack of chocolate, one tube of cheese spread, one tube of condensed milk, four packs of instant coffee, six Oxo cubes, 8 oz. wholemeal biscuits, one box of matches and a lightweight cooking stove and saucepan.

Before rejecting such advice as silly fuss, one should reflect that in recent years in Britain about twenty people have died each summer from exposure on hills and mountains. Most have been teenagers, often attempting over-ambitious programmes.

Outside Britain the same dangers are found, but the higher the mountains the less forgiving they are. With increasing altitude there is a bigger difference between daytime and night temperatures, and the cold nights are a real hazard for a party delayed by a trivial accident.

Mountain sickness

Until very recently it was possible to reach high mountains only by a slow approach on foot, and this necessarily gave the body time to adjust to the change in atmospheric pressure that occurs with altitude. Now, however, tourists and others can reach areas at 12,000 feet (3,600 metres) or more within twenty-four hours of leaving Europe; and it has become clear that such rapid change in altitude may cause serious and even fatal lung disease. The condition is unknown below 9,000 feet and rare below 12,000 feet. Recently a lot of detailed information on the condition has come from studies of troops in the Indian army, for whom it is a major problem when soldiers are moved from the plains to the Himalayas.

At high altitudes the lowered atmospheric pressure reduces the availability of oxygen. The breathing rate has to be increased in order to maintain normal oxygen levels in the blood; and this increased breathing rate eliminates more than usual carbon dioxide from the body, so changing the acidity of the blood. This causes symptoms such as headache, sickness, loss of appetite and difficulty in sleeping.

These symptoms are unpleasant, though not in themselves dangerous: but a minority of sufferers from mountain sickness also develop sudden difficulty in breathing. This is due to flooding of the lungs with fluid, which for reasons not fully understood diffuses out of the bloodstream into the airspaces. Without treatment, this pulmonary oedema may be fatal quickly. Emergency treatment includes oxygen and drugs which increase the flow of urine, but the only certain remedy is a rapid return to low altitude. Current recommendations by mountain safety organizations include the provision of stretchers and oxygen at strategic points at high altitude.

Acute pulmonary oedema may develop very suddenly without any other symptoms of mountain sickness. Surprisingly, the persons most at risk seem to be muscular men in their teens or early twenties, who are in good physical condition. Exposure to cold seems to be a possible precipitating factor: deaths have been reported on several occasions in climbers who developed pulmonary oedema after a swim in a mountain lake.

As with so many conditions, the only reliable protection is prevention. Acclimatization to altitude takes time, and it is unwise to climb above 12,000 feet without having spent at least two weeks at heights of 6,000 feet or more. If this is impossible, then at the very least every climber should take with him some tablets of the drug frusemide. Should pulmonary oedema develop – and there is no mistaking the severe breathlessness *at rest*, combined with cough and mental confusion – then two 40-mg. tablets of frusemide every four hours may be life-saving, giving valuable time for the victim to be carried down to a safe altitude. It is now recognized that high altitude may affect other parts of the body, such as the eyes, brain or kidneys, but less commonly than the lungs.

Sailing and swimming

Most of the hazards of water-borne leisure activities are well known – yet several hundred persons drown every year in Britain and thousands in North America. Non-swimmers still go out in small boats without wearing a life-jacket and indifferent swimmers ignore warning flags on beaches.

Recent research by naval experts and others, particularly on the importance of water temperature on survival, is not yet widely known. But investigation of shipwreck disasters such as the fire on the cruise liner *Lakonia* has shown that in European waters most deaths are due to cold rather than to drowning. Immersion in water at about 4°C. causes rapid cooling of the body, and consciousness may be lost within fifteen minutes or less. In really cold water such as that around Iceland survival for more than a few minutes is impossible without protective clothing.

The surprising result of research studies has been the demonstration that anyone plunged into cold water reduces his chance of survival by swimming. Vigorous muscular exertion uses up the body's stores of energy rapidly; and the rapid circulation of blood through the skin speeds the cooling process. In contrast, the shipwreck survivor who lies quietly in his life-jacket or simply treads water to stay afloat can conserve energy, while the blood-vessels in the skin can shut down, so minimizing the cooling effect. Therefore anyone unfortunate enough to be on a sinking ship or yacht should put on several layers of thick clothing and a life-jacket and delay entering the water until the last possible safe moment.

For the same reason, anyone in a small sailing dinghy which capsizes should stay with the upturned boat rather than attempt to swim to the shore. Getting on to the boat, even if it is swamped, will preserve body heat, and hence increase one's chances of survival.

Water-skiing

While most people recognize that they should equip themselves properly and receive expert instruction for snow-skiing, a much more casual attitude is taken to water-skiing. Holidaymakers offered thirty minutes' free water-skiing instruction happily take up the offer, dressing only in bathing trunks. In fact as with any other high-speed sport proper instruction and gear are needed.

Each year cases are reported of internal injury to inexperienced water-skiers who come off the skis at speed: water can be forced into the body via the rectum or vagina. This does not occur, of course, if pants are worn which cannot be penetrated by water, and these should be used by all novice water-skiers.

The other common medical consequence of water-skiing by a novice is a painful swelling of the tendons at the wrist (de Quervain's disease, tenosynovitis) caused by the tension on the arms. This is a painful condition, but it is resolved within a week or two if the muscles and tendons are rested.

Chapter 6

TRAVEL

I F 'travelling is the ruin of all happiness', as Fanny Burney claimed, it is a hazard to which few of our ancestors exposed themselves. As recently as the nineteenth century most people never left the country of their birth and a journey of a hundred miles was a considerable expedition. Indeed travelling was thought to be such an unnatural activity that the disease tabes dorsalis, which often affected sailors, commercial travellers and long-distance engine-drivers, was thought by medical authorities to be caused by the long distances they covered in their work – only later was it found to be a late complication of syphilis.

In fact there are several medical hazards of travel, and of these the most serious is the risk of acquiring a disease which does not occur in one's home country. About eight million Britons go abroad for their holidays each year, while others have to travel for business reasons. Jet travel is so fast that it is only too easy for a traveller to have been home for a week or more before any symptoms develop of an illness acquired abroad, and doctors are constantly being reminded that they must ask their patients about recent journeys overseas if they are not to miss cases of tropical disease.

MALARIA

Probably the most dangerous disease for international travellers is malaria. Several thousand cases occur each year in Europeans returning from Africa, Asia and South America; and since symptoms may be delayed for weeks and months it is easy for a doctor to miss the diagnosis. In recent years the number of cases reported each year in Britain has risen steadily, probably as a result of increased business and holiday travel outside Europe. In the last year for which detailed figures are available, 1973, the 541 cases were made up of 102 immigrants, 187 tourists, eighty-eight long-term residents abroad, eleven servicemen and air-crew, thirty-seven businessmen, and eight children visiting parents abroad. The circumstances were not reported in 108 cases. There were five deaths, and in these cases it appeared that precautions had not been taken against malaria. The time interval between return to the United Kingdom and the onset of malaria was less than six months in 84 per cent of cases, but there were a few where the interval was over one year.

Malaria is a feverish illness caused by several species of organisms called plasmodia. It is acquired only by the bite of an infected mosquito of a particular type. (The one exception is transfusion of blood taken from a donor with malaria, but this is extremely uncommon.) The life-cycle of malaria parasites is complicated: they multiply within the red cells in the bloodstream of an infected individual, but part of the life-cycle has to be completed inside the body of the mosquito.

The characteristic feature of malaria is the regular pattern of the fever. In the most common type, benign tertian malaria, the parasites enter red blood cells, where they take seventy-two hours to complete a single cycle of multiplication. The blood cell then bursts, releasing a new generation of parasites into the bloodstream. This seventy-two-hour cycle produces a sudden rise in temperature to as high as 107°F. every third day, coinciding with the release of a new generation of parasites.

About a quarter of the cases occurring in Britain are of the malignant tertian form of the disease, by far the most dangerous type. Malignant malaria can cause blockage in vital blood-vessels supplying the brain and so cause a stroke in a young healthy adult.

Unfortunately many people who travel to parts of the world where they may pick up malaria are unaware of the risk. A single bite from an infected mosquito is enough to transmit malaria, and such a bite may occur during a refuelling stop on a flight from one non-malarious country to another. Since no one can guarantee that they will avoid being bitten by a mosquito the only safe policy is for everyone passing through malarious areas to take preventive treatment.

Reliable information on which countries are free from the risk of malaria is published by the World Health Organization and updated frequently.* There is no risk of malaria in Europe (except for the eastern tip of Greece), the USA, Canada, Australia, New Zealand or Japan. Almost every part of Africa still has malaria, including Morocco, Tunisia and Egypt; so does Central and South America, India and the Middle and Far East.

Persons travelling to or through these areas should take preventive treatment. All that is required is a once-weekly dose of pyrimethamine, but this must start a week before reaching the malarious area and must be continued for a month after leaving it. Perhaps a more realistic alternative is that used by the British Armed Forces, who argue that once-a-week dosage is easily forgotten and recommend instead one tablet a day of an alternative drug, proguanil.

Quite a number of the recent cases in Britain have been children of Asians returning to their home countries for holidays. The parents may very well have built up immunity in early adult life, but the children born in Britain have never had any need to acquire it.

Anyone who has been in a malarious area should tell his doctor should he or she develop any illness within a year of the trip. The diagnosis is not obvious unless suspected, and most British general practitioners have never seen a case.

* *Information on Malaria Risk for International Travellers*, obtainable from WHO, 1211, Geneva 27, Switzerland.

TRAVELLER'S DIARRHOEA

Probably the commonest medical problem for the international traveller is an acute attack of diarrhoea that occurs within a few days of arrival. There are countless names for this complaint: gyppy tummy, Aden Gut, Basra belly, Delhi belly, Hong Kong dog, Montezuma's revenge, the Aztec two-step and turista; and the very number of these terms demonstrates the worldwide distribution of the disorder. It seems particularly prevalent in the Middle East, Mexico and North Africa, but it may be troublesome in any part of the world.

What distinguishes traveller's diarrhoea from other forms of gastrointestinal disturbance is that it affects only newcomers to an area: the established members of the community are not affected. A series of careful studies have been done in recent years of servicemen travelling abroad. In 1967, for example, it was reported that half the American servicemen arriving in Vietnam had an attack of diarrhoea within their first two months in the country. Three years later a group of British servicemen were flown out to Aden at short notice and of 540 soldiers thirty-eight developed acute diarrhoea in the first fourteen days.

Bacteriological tests were done on the British soldiers and these showed no trace of any of the well-known organisms responsible for food poisoning: but the tests also showed that all the soldiers taken ill had in their intestines a particular strain of the bacterium *Escherichia coli*. This is one of the bacteria – commensals – that are usually found in the intestines, where they assist in the digestion of food and cause no harm. It seems that in each part of the world the local inhabitants have learnt to live with a particular strain of *Escherichia coli*, and that a traveller who eats food contaminated with a strain that is new to him is likely to have an attack of diarrhoea. Recently laboratory tests have become widely available of 'typing' these bacteria; and it seems, for example, that the strain responsible for outbreaks in Aden, 0148K H28, does not occur at all in Britain.

Further confirmation that traveller's diarrhoea is caused by unfamiliar bacteria comes from its prevention by anti-bacterial drugs. Over 1,000 BOAC personnel and their families took part in one recent study of this form of treatment: compared with those who took no medicines, those who took antibiotic Streptotriad tablets had fewer attacks of diarrhoea and the attacks they had were less severe.

It has been calculated that if a family of four spends a two-week holiday abroad on average one member will have an attack of traveller's diarrhoea during that time, so there seems some justification for taking precautionary treatment with Streptotriad. Another popular but unproved remedy is Enterovioform (clioquinol), but doubts have been raised about the safety of this compound (see p. 97). On the other hand anyone going to a new country for a lengthy stay would be ill-advised to take antibiotics indefinitely: much better to get used to the new bacteria even if this means a few days' discomfort.

CHOLERA, TYPHOID AND PLAGUE

To the traveller of the nineteenth and early twentieth century travel abroad carried a genuine risk of death from one of the classic killers – cholera, typhoid and plague. All three diseases still exist, but the World Health Organization now maintains an effective surveillance system and can give reliable information on which countries have active disease at any given time. Immunization is available against all three diseases, though the protection offered is not as complete as that given against smallpox by vaccination.

Cholera has recently been spreading west from India and the Middle East. In 1973 there was a serious outbreak in Naples, and no holiday resort on the Mediterranean can now be assumed to be free from some risk of the disease. Cholera is an intestinal infection caught by eating food or drinking water contaminated by infected human excreta. Clearly, therefore, the best precaution against the disease is to drink only 'safe' water, avoiding wells, standpipes and springs, and to resist the temptation of meals of uncooked seafood or ice-cream made in a back kitchen. A healthy adult who catches cholera should not die if proper medical treatment is available: immunization gives useful protection for a few months only.

Typhoid is more prevalent in Europe than cholera: every year a few cases occur among British travellers to Spain and southern France. Like cholera, it is an intestinal disease caught from infected food or drink. There the resemblance ends, however. Cholera causes profuse diarrhoea and the disease develops within hours or at most a day or two of infection. Typhoid is a generalized illness (p. 75) and its onset may be delayed for two to three weeks after infection. Most holiday-makers who acquire typhoid fall ill only on their return home. Typhoid is a serious disease: of the 200 or so cases that occur each year in Britain a few are fatal. Immunization greatly reduces the risk of a severe attack of the disease, but to be effective two injections of the vaccine are needed with an interval of at least ten days between them.

Plague is now only a problem in the Far East. It is a form of blood-poisoning due to bacteria which are transmitted by blood-sucking fleas. Antibiotic treatment is effective if given early in the disease, and immunization gives good protection.

SMALLPOX

In 1975 the World Health Organization announced that it expected smallpox to be eliminated within one or two years at most. During the course of the year India, Pakistan and Bangladesh reported themselves free of the disease, and by the beginning of 1976 the only country in which cases were still being notified was Ethiopia. Vigilance will be maintained for some years yet, however: and there is always a possibility of a repetition of the outbreak in London in 1973, in which three cases were acquired from smallpox kept in a research laboratory.

The eradication of smallpox has been due to vaccination campaigns, and not unreasonably many countries insist on evidence of recent vaccination in travellers arriving from the East. In general vaccination is no longer required for travellers within Europe and North America. Within Britain vaccination is no longer recommended for children, since the disease is now so rare that the very small risk of complications from the vaccination can no longer be justified. Indeed, this risk is probably greater than the risk of getting smallpox.

WORMS AND FLUKES

The lack of adequate sewage-disposal systems found in so many underdeveloped countries – especially those with tropical and equatorial climates – encourages transmission of parasitic intestinal worms including tapeworms, roundworms and threadworms (p. 78). Such parasites are also prevalent wherever human excrement is used as a fertilizer. Punctilious attention to cleanliness in the preparation of food is essential if infection is to be avoided, though in practice mild infections often cause no symptoms. Nevertheless, Europeans are often distressed if they notice worms or worm segments in their faeces. Treatment is simple and effective.

In much of the tropical world anyone who goes barefoot risks acquiring infection with hookworm – small bloodsucking worms that live in the upper intestine and can cause profound anaemia.

Schistosomiasis is one of the last remaining medical challenges among infectious diseases. It affects hundreds of millions of people in Africa and the Far East, causing chronic illness and death. Schistosoma are worms (strictly flukes) which live in the blood-vessels around the liver and intestines in one form of the disease and around the bladder in the other form. Each worm may spend many years inside the body, laying millions of eggs which are passed out with the excreta or the urine.

The life-cycle of schistosoma is complicated: the eggs passed in human excreta hatch in fresh water, where the larvae die unless they find a particular kind of snail, in which further stages of development occur. Man becomes affected by walking or swimming in water containing diseased snails: and in practice this means almost any freshwater lake or stream in endemic areas. The disease is treatable, but can be cured completely only if detected at an early stage. Public health campaigns have mostly been directed against the snails, with some success; but recently the condition has spread to some islands in the eastern Caribbean including St Lucia and Guadaloupe.

INSECT BITES

Insects sometimes spoil an otherwise perfect holiday, since they are most numerous in summer weather and often breed close to salt or fresh water. Mosquitoes, midges and gnats are found in all parts of the world: oddly enough they are particularly troublesome in the extremes of climate, so the Briton who goes north to Scotland or Scandinavia is just as troubled by them as those who go to the Mediterranean. Insects tend to bite at dusk, and the wise traveller dresses to cover his arms, ankles and feet before settling down to an evening drink. Annoyingly for the tourist, local inhabitants are far less troubled by insect bites than newcomers: again, this is a question of immunity, which takes time to develop. Both locals and tourists are at risk from insect-borne infections, however. These vary in each part of the world: in addition to malaria insect-borne diseases include yellow fever, sandfly fever, dengue and encephalitis of various kinds. Vaccination is available against some of these diseases and is advisable if an infected area is to be visited.

The other well-known disease transmitted by insects is typhus (a serious illness with a fever, rash and disturbed consciousness). This, however, is acquired from body lice and is unlikely to trouble the tourist.

SNAKES AND SCORPIONS

Snakes, scorpions and spiders such as the black widow are among the major anxieties of parents taking their children to tropical countries. Most such animals are nocturnal, seeking the shade by day. They may attack if disturbed by someone lifting a stone; and clearly it is hazardous to walk through undergrowth barefoot or in sandals. Deaths from poisonous bites are, however, rare except in India, where several hundred of the rural population die from snake bites each year.

Mortality from snake bite is variable. The most dangerous seems to be the Taiwan krait, for which a death rate of 20 per cent has been reported recently. Cobras are dangerous – mortality rate 7 per cent – followed by sea snakes. Viper bites cause death far less often, and even species with a sinister reputation such as the Malayan pit viper are associated with a death rate of only 1 per cent.

Viper bites typically cause severe damage to the skin and muscle at the site of the puncture wound, and this local necrosis comes on within a few hours of the bite. In contrast, the dangerous cobras, kraits and mambas cause nervous paralysis, and death may ensue from paralysis of the breathing muscles or from a direct poisonous effect on the heart.

Less than half of all those bitten by poisonous snakes are in fact poisoned – often no venom is injected. Since treatment with antivenom has its dangers it is best reserved for those victims who show unequivocal signs of poisoning. The important thing is not to move the part of the body that has been bitten.

HEPATITIS

Hepatitis – inflammation of the liver causing jaundice – is a virus disease that is one of the few serious health hazards for the European visitor to an undeveloped country. There are two forms of the disease, hepatitis A and B, caused by different viruses.

Hepatitis A is the common infectious jaundice, formerly a prevalent childhood illness in Britain. Usually mild, the illness is transmitted by faulty personal hygiene: the infected person passes the virus in his excreta, and new infections are acquired via contaminated food and water. The disease is more prevalent in countries with inadequate sewage systems.

Hepatitis B, also known as serum hepatitis, is a more serious illness with a considerable mortality. For many years it was thought that hepatitis B could only be transmitted by blood-to-blood contact such as by a blood transfusion from an infected person, among drug addicts by sharing a syringe or needle, or by amateur tattooing. More refined tests have shown, however, that the high prevalence of the condition in tropical countries means that it should be added to the list of diseases transmitted by blood-sucking insects such as mosquitoes. Furthermore, there is now conclusive evidence that hepatitis B can be transmitted during sexual intercourse — there is a high incidence of infections among prostitutes and homosexuals. Anyone travelling outside Europe and North America should consider a precautionary injection of human gammaglobulin, which gives reasonable protection against hepatitis A for up to six months.

SUNBURN AND SUNSTROKE

Anyone with only a week or two in the sun likes to make the best possible use of it: so it is sad that so many tourists spoil the early days of their holidays by over-exposure to the sun. Someone used only to British sun cannot safely sunbathe for over ten minutes on the first day on the shore of the Mediterranean in summer. It takes at least forty-eight hours for a tan to start, and during this time the skin must be protected.

Sunburn may be unpleasant, but sunstroke may be dangerous. Just as it takes time to acclimatize to altitude, so the body needs time to adjust to a rise in the air temperature. Until this internal thermostat has been reset a combination if intense heat and physical exertion will lead to loss of enormous volumes of sweat. Unless this is replaced – and that means replacement of salt as well as water – collapse is inevitable. Tourists who play strenuous games such as tennis or go climbing hills in the midday heat have only themselves to blame if they become dizzy and faint.

CULTURAL SHOCK

Cultural shock is a term used by American psychologists to describe a not uncommon response by anyone who spends any length of time in an unfamiliar culture. Indeed it is argued that this psychological phenomenon is experienced in some degree by all persons who live (not just travel) for extended periods in a culture and environment different from their own.

Characteristically the effect of cultural shock is to induce depression associated with profound disgust for the people, customs and values of the host country. Social orientation is lost, and the sufferer may develop feelings of persecution: every trivial mishap is blamed on the stupidity and uncivilized behaviour of the natives. If the condition goes unrecognized for what it is – an abnormal mental response to the stress of acclimatization to a foreign environment – it may precipitate further problems such as excessive drinking.

The new arrival in a country is usually so excited and interested by its contrasts with his own background that he is protected from the hazard of cultural shock. Instead, his reaction is critical of other foreigners who criticize native behaviour and customs. This is a dangerous sign, according to American authorities on the condition. Once a newcomer has convinced himself that he possesses a better mental attitude than residents of long standing he is almost certain to develop cultural shock, for eventually he will be forced to change his attitude to one closer to the norm, and this change is likely to prove difficult to accept psychologically.

TRAVELLER'S PSYCHOSIS

If cultural shock is almost inevitable for anyone who changes cultures, then traveller's psychosis is rare. The condition – also called 'travel syndrome' – is an acute mental breakdown that comes on after two or three days' continuous travel. It is almost always a lone traveller who is affected; and often he has been in two minds about making the journey. While travelling he has eaten irregularly, slept little and drunk too much alcohol.

The illness begins suddenly with hallucinations and delusions, and this may involve mistaken beliefs that the traveller is being laughed at by locals or is under suspicion of crime or of spreading venereal disease. Sometimes these beliefs lead the traveller to make unprovoked assaults or to attempt spectacular escapes by, for example, leaping out of the door of a moving train. The condition generally settles with rest and sedation – but this presupposes that sympathetic medical attention is available in the country and district where the illness develops.

CHANGES IN THE BODY CLOCK

Most people are now aware that rapid travel over long distances may lead to considerable disturbances of natural rhythms of sleep, digestion, etc. This effect is known as disturbance of the circadian rhythms or body clock, and has been the subject of enormous amounts of research in recent years, particularly in the context of space travel.

Circadian rhythms – so called because they are based on a period of about one day – are found in all living organisms, plant or animal. In man there is a regular variation with the time of day in body temperature, heart rate, sweating, production of urine by the kidneys, digestion, hunger and, most prominently, sleep. We are all familiar with the difficulty of sleeping during the day even if we have been forced to stay awake all night. There is clearly an evolutionary advantage in the body being able to switch into low gear during sleep.

The timing mechanism of biological rhythms is still unknown. It is not simply a matter of light and darkness, as has been shown by experiments in which volunteers have spent long periods either in artificial light or deep underground. When a man is separated from the natural rhythm of day and night and is also deprived of any timing mechanism his body continues to function on the same twenty-four-hour cycle. The length of the cycle is usually not quite twenty-four hours; most people 'running free' maintain a day of between twenty-three hours and twenty-five hours. Conversely, in an artificial environment (such as a polar research base during the six months of winter) men function quite happily on a day as short as twenty hours or as long as twenty-eight, but the internal clock cannot adapt beyond these limits.

Practical problems with circadian rhythms occur whenever the body clock is thrown out of time by a change in routine. In its simpler form this happens with shift-working, when factory or hospital staff may spend alternate weeks on 'days' and 'nights'. Experience during the Second World War showed that most shift-workers take several days to adjust their internal clocks to a new routine of sleeping, eating and activity. Until this change is made the worker feels sleepy during his shift, but on his return to bed finds his mind alert – and his stomach hungry, his kidneys producing urine and his bowels active. For this reason experienced shift-workers prefer to switch from days to nights as infrequently as possible.

An air traveller who moves through several time zones is in the same position as a worker changing his shift. The businessman who travels from London to China undergoes a ten-hour change, so that when the hotel serves breakfast at 9 a.m. his internal clock is still set at 11 p.m. and is switching the body into low gear for a period of sleep. Practical experience with air travel has shown that most people can adjust their internal clock to a new cycle no faster than one hour a day, and there is some evidence that solitary travellers adjust more slowly than groups. Since each 15° of longitude travelled corresponds to a time-switch of one hour (15° corresponds to one time-zone – the band of land in which all clocks show the same time), a simple calculation can be done to estimate the number of days needed to acclimatize to a change in geographical location.

For practical purposes the problem is only important with air travel, since even a fast passenger liner rarely covers more than 30° of longitude in a day except near to one or other pole, and even long-distance trains do not traverse more than two or three time-zones in a day.

A rapid journey through five or more time-zones is certain to disturb the body's internal clock; but it may also cause quite alarming symptoms. Anyone who refuses to accept the inevitability of a disturbance of his biological rhythms and attempts to fulfil a strenuous programme of engagements is likely to become confused and disorientated – and his judgement may become very shaky (p. 19).

MEDICAL TREATMENT ABROAD

Few other countries have a comprehensive National Health Service like that in Britain. Medical treatment may be very expensive, even for a comparatively trivial condition such as a broken arm or an operation for appendicitis. A traveller seriously injured in a motor accident or needing hospital treatment for a major condition such as a coronary thrombosis or a ruptured duodenal ulcer might easily face a bill for more than £1,000.

Within the EEC medical treatment is part of social security insurance; the patient pays fees to the doctor or hospital and is reimbursed for most of the bill by the insurance institutions. United Kingdom citizens and their dependents are usually eligible for these benefits on a reciprocal basis: full details are available from the Department of Health (Leaflet SA 28, forms E 111 and CM 1). These social security payments will reimburse a patient for at least 70 per cent of the cost of treatment, provided that the doctor that he chooses does not charge more than the standard tariff. In popular holiday resorts it is unwise to assume that the doctors will necessarily stick to tariff charges.

Medical insurance may, indeed, be a wise investment for the EEC traveller: it is essential for anyone going further afield.

SELF-TREATMENT

Not unnaturally, many holiday travellers prefer to treat their own minor ailments rather than look for a doctor and then try to explain their symptoms in an unfamiliar language. There is an understandable temptation to go to a chemist's shop and look for or ask for a 'bottle of cough medicine' or some skin cream.

Self-treatment abroad may be dangerous. Over-the-counter medicines are legally controlled much more rigorously in Britain than elsewhere, and in most of Europe highly dangerous drugs can be bought without prescription. One example of the sort of tragedy that can occur was the death of a young English woman in 1972. On holiday in Spain she developed a cough and bought a bottle of cough medicine at the local chemist's shop. This contained a powerful antibiotic, chloramphenicol, obtainable only on prescription in Britain and little used by doctors because of its known dangerous side-effects. Some weeks after her return to Britain the woman developed a fatal blood disease, a direct consequence of the chloramphenicol.

Self-treatment is a perfectly reasonable policy, but it is safer to get medical advice on the choice of drugs and to include them in the holiday luggage.

Chapter 7

OCCUPATION

THE Industrial Revolution had appalling effects on the health of the new class of urban industrial workers in Britain. Blake's dark, Satanic mills were subject to no form of State inspection, and the combination of uncontrolled pollution, dangerous machinery and long working days led to high rates of industrial disease and death. The terrible conditions aroused the conscience of reformers, and by the middle of the nineteenth century the more obvious occupational hazards had been recognized. The next half century was spent in eliminating these dangers, improving ventilation, reducing working hours, and generally improving the lot of workers. Much was achieved by industrial legislation; other improvements in safety came from the introduction of more refined industrial processes. Most of the terrible occupational diseases – such as 'hatters' shakes' (mercury poisoning affecting the brain in workmen felting hats), or 'phossy jaw' (destruction of the jawbone by white phosphorus in match-workers) – were relegated to the textbook by the beginning of the twentieth century.

Occupational diseases are still an important cause of illness and premature death, however. Part of the explanation lies in old lessons forgotten or risks inherent in the job – usually accidents or dust; but there is also a steady succession of newly recognized industrial diseases. Sometimes no one has noticed a connection between the disease and the occupation – as in the case of a form of liver cancer only recently shown to occur in men working on the manufacture of the plastic polyvinylchloride. New industries also create their own diseases, and management in industry has now learnt to be constantly on the look-out for these. A typical recent example of a new hazard occurred on the introduction of biological washing powders, which contain enzymes to digest proteins derived from a micro-organism called *Bacillus subtilis.* Soon after they had been introduced some workers began to complain of chest troubles – cough, shortness of breath and chest pain. Special tests showed that a few of them were sensitive to dusts containing extracts of *Bacillus subtilis*, and new processes have now been devised to minimize exposure to these.

Once such a new disease is identified the Inspector of Factories should act swiftly to abolish the risks. In theory at least, all serious and fatal accidents and sixteen different types of industrial diseases have to be notified under the Factories Act, and there are similar provisions for mineworkers and quarrymen. Unfortunately the emphasis put on prevention and safety precautions varies markedly from industry to industry and there are also variations within each industry. Small firms employing only a few men often operate on margins which encourage them to cut corners if money can be saved.

Occasionally also new techniques of analysis have revealed risks in occupations which employed too few workers for the hazard to be obvious. The Oxford Record Linkage Study collects a unique mass of data from all patients in the area served by the hospital board, whether they have been seen by the general practitioner, hospital or community health services, and analyses these using a computer. One of the first results of this research was to show a remarkably high incidence of a rare type of cancer of the sinuses around the nose, principally affecting woodworkers in the High Wycombe furniture industry. Although the numbers were relatively small (twenty-nine woodworkers out of a total of thirty-five patients), the incidence was comparatively high – roughly the same as that of breast cancer in women or lung cancer in men in the general population.

Further research by the Oxford medical team showed that similar workers elsewhere in Britain also run this risk, that it probably existed as early as 1920 and at least as recently as 1940, and that on average the tumour takes thirty-nine years to develop. Upholsterers, French-polishers and varnishers were found to run no increased risk of developing the tumour; since their work is usually done in separate, dust-free shops, the hazard is probably contained in wood dust or particles of other material associated with it. Moreover, wood dust was found to be deposited on particular areas of the lining of the nose, and this showed microscopical changes suggesting precancer. Professor Acheson and his colleagues suggested that the government should classify this type of cancer as an industrial disease, and this was done in 1969 (a year after their report). Research is continuing – in particular to see if the introduction of exhaust ventilation into the factories in the 1940s had abolished the risk.

DIFFERENTIAL RISKS

The main difficulty in deciding whether some illnesses are commoner in some occupations than others is that most of our statistics are based on death (mortality) rather than illness (morbidity). Most experts agree that mortality rates probably underestimate morbidity rates; for example, a man may have disabling chronic bronchitis for years which does not shorten life and may not even eventually be recorded on his death certificate. Records for sickness absence from work are available (p. 147), but, though these are classified by diagnosis, they do not mention occupation.

Deaths and serious injuries due to accidents in premises subject to the Factories Act have to be notified to HM Inspector of Factories – as do cases of industrial poisoning or disease – and these are published in an annual report. Other reports giving similar details are produced by the Inspector of Mines and Quarries and the Registrar General of Shipping and Seamen. Nevertheless, the main basis of estimating the connection between occupations and particular types of illness remains the Registrar General's *Occupational Mortality Tables*, which are published only every ten years, and then relating to a period ten years before the date of the report. The most recent report was published in December 1971 and dealt with deaths occurring in 1961. This breaks down statistics on people by their social class (I, professional, to V, unskilled occupations) and by their occupations or that of their husbands (twenty-seven orders and 340 categories). The main index used is the standardized mortality ratio (SMR), which is the ratio of the deaths noted in a particular group, divided by the number of deaths expected in the general population between fifteen and sixty-four years old multiplied by 100. An SMR of 100 is average: high-risk occupations have SMR values above that figure, while 'safe' jobs such as schoolteaching have a value of less than 100.

These figures are certainly extremely valuable but one of the drawbacks of the report – as the Registrar General points out – is that men in strenuous work such as mining tend to move into lighter work as they get older, and the cause of death may be linked with the wrong occupation. Other sources of error include the preference of healthy (or less healthy) men for particular jobs, and the movement of ill men from one job into another, but there is nothing that can be done to correct these sources of error with the present arrangements. Despite all this, however, these statistics do show some sort of picture of occupational hazards of both morbidity and mortality.

COAL-MINERS

Face workers in coal-mining have one of the highest standardized mortality rates on record. For all causes this is 180, and for several individual diseases the rate is considerably higher than average; for example, cancer at all sites, heart disease and nephritis. Nevertheless, four causes of death stand out prominently: bronchitis; accidents; respiratory tuberculosis, with occupational disease of the lung; and occupational pneumoconiosis – at SMRs of 293, 522, 2,650, and 3,500 respectively.

Despite the high mortality from accidents among miners

there has been a steady fall in the number of accidents reported at the coal-face in the last few years, partly owing to the decline in numbers of coal-face workers but probably also to greater safety consciousness and to the use of new techniques which reduce working hazards. Thus in 1972 sixty-four people were killed and 519 seriously injured in coal-mines – seven and sixty-nine, respectively, of these occurring on the surface. This was a fall in the accident rate of 0·01 per 100,000 man-shifts for the previous year. Even so, a total of almost 59,000 injuries involved absences for over three days, and, although accidents at the coal-face declined, the number of surface accidents did not fall, while those involving haulage and transport actually rose. Thus in 1972 falls of ground (which until 1968 was the principal cause of all major accidents) caused a third of the deaths or serious injuries underground, less than those due to haulage and transport, and much the same as those due to miscellaneous causes, including machinery, explosions and shaft accidents. In his 1972 report the Chief Inspector of Mines and Quarries commented that 'it is disturbing to note the frequency with which "Failure to comply with recognized good practice" is quoted', and suggested in particular that haulage methods should be reviewed and corrected. There are more underground haulage accidents on the roads than at the coal-face and most arise from incidents involving tub and mine cars, roadway conveyors and locomotives. At the surface, too, accidents involving vehicles and machines are common causes.

Pneumoconiosis

The Report of the Chief Inspector of Mines also cites the incidence of new cases of pneumoconiosis diagnosed in coal-miners. Pneumoconiosis is defined as a permanent disease which results from the accumulation of mineral dust in the lungs and the reaction of the tissues to it, but not including bronchitis or emphysema (over-inflation of the lung). If somebody consistently breathes air containing suspended particles measuring between 0·5 and 5/1,000 mm. in diameter there is a good chance that these will settle in the smallest air passages or air sacs. Here they may provoke the lung tissue to form nodules of scar tissue, up to 5 mm. in diameter, and, in relation to these, tiny blisters containing air may develop (a condition called focal emphysema). When enough of these nodules are present they appear on an X-ray film of the chest as a fine stippled effect throughout the lungs. This appearance is known as simple pneumoconiosis, and is classified into four separate grades as the amount of stippling in the chest X-ray film progressively increases. Some people, however, also eventually develop large masses, usually in the upper part of both lungs, which may get progressively bigger and spread to the rest of the lungs. This, known as complicated pneumoconiosis, is classified into three grades of severity, and is probably due to an abnormal reaction to an infection with tuberculosis in somebody who already has the simple type of the disease.

Coal-miners' pneumoconiosis seems to be caused by pure coal dust (and has become particularly common since machines have been used for cutting the coal) and not by silica or some other material present in the coal. Most cases affect coal-face workers, but it also occurs in people such as dockers who handle coal; for this reason it is also called coal-workers' pneumoconiosis. Pneumoconiosis is, however, commoner with some types of coal than others, occurring more frequently in men working with anthracite than with bituminous coals. With 626 new cases (2·3 per 1,000 men employed) in 1972 the incidence is now falling, but 10,000 of the 280,000 coal-miners in Britain receive benefit for chest troubles attributed to their work by the Pneumoconiosis Medical Panels and the disease still causes 900 deaths a year.

Much of our knowledge of pneumoconiosis and its effect has come from the National Coal Board's Medical Units and especially the Medical Research Council Pneumoconiosis

Research Unit, established in Cardiff in 1944. But despite a lot of research there is still considerable controversy not only about how the changes in the lungs are produced but also about their effects on health and the expectation of life. Symptoms – shortness of breath, loss of weight, loss of energy – do not necessarily correspond in severity with laboratory evidence of impaired breathing. Miners with or without pneumoconiosis often have bronchitis, which also causes breathlessness, and this condition is common enough in all industrial workers, whatever their job – particularly if they smoke heavily. Hence a doctor may find it very difficult to decide how much of a specific miner's ill-health is directly due to his work, and how much to his smoking and to life in the cold, damp environment of a Welsh valley. Laboratory measurements show that the lungs in simple pneumoconiosis are not quite as efficient as normal, whether the miner has symptoms or not, and that this reduction is linked to his age and to the amount of dust to which he has been exposed. Every year between 1 and 2 per cent of miners with simple pneumoconiosis develop the complicated type, in which breathlessness is usually severe, increasing in direct proportion to the degree of abnormality in the chest X-ray film.

Despite the controversy, from the practical viewpoint, the National Coal Board spends £3½ million a year on medical research into pneumoconiosis. It maintains a full-time occupational health service, and every miner has a regular chest X-ray examination from a mobile unit which visits the pits periodically. The aim is to spot any serious progression in the pneumoconiosis in any individual miner and to remove him from heavy exposure to coal dust straightaway.

During the same visit the mobile unit assesses the methods of dust suppression being used. New standards for dust levels were laid down in 1970 to try to reduce pneumoconiosis. Dust suppression is carried out principally by efficient ventilation and extensive use of water in cutting and drilling operations. On occasions when the production of dust is unavoidable, face-masks are used.

Miners with pneumoconiosis are compensated according to the degree of disability they experience, X-ray films being used only to diagnose the condition and not to assess its effects. Even so, these judgements are often extraordinarily difficult: the Pneumoconiosis Medical Panels have to decide what proportion of a man's disability is due to pneumoconiosis, bronchitis and emphysema. If a miner is judged to have at least 50 per cent disability then any disability due to chronic bronchitis or emphysema is taken into account in the amount of compensation awarded. But if his disability is less than this amount, then added disability from these conditions is inadmissible. Understandably, this ruling is attacked by some doctors and most miners, though only 4 per cent of them need to be paid compensation.

Other conditions

Miners can suffer from several other less serious conditions linked with their occupation, including 'beat knee', 'beat elbow', athlete's foot, Weil's disease, heat cramp and nystagmus. 'Beat' knee and elbow are the names given to inflammation of the skin and the bursae (fluid-filled sacs) over the joints. In lying down or kneeling to cut the coal a miner may put great pressure on the skin around the joints (up to 200 lb. per square inch for the knee). This can cause small blood-vessels to burst and bleed into the bursa, which eventually becomes filled with scar tissue. The pressure on the skin may cause cracks and cuts in it and allow bacteria to enter with inflammation of the tissues under the surface. Similar infections of the hand cause the 'beat hand' of miners. The problem of the beat disorders can be tackled in two ways: by devising improved pads to distribute the pressure on the knees more evenly, and by providing pit baths for the miners after every shift to minimize the amount of infection. Pit baths themselves, however, may be responsible for transmitting the fungus of athlete's foot, which is present on the floors of the changing-rooms and showers.

Weil's disease, which may seriously affect the liver and kidneys, is due to a micro-organism commonly present in rat's urine (p. 175). The declining use of ponies in the mines has been followed by a reduction in the number of rats and in the incidence of Weil's disease among coal-miners. Heat cramps occur in men who have lost large amounts of salt in the sweat (up to 1 oz. in a shift) and drunk excessive amounts of fluid, a combination of events which results in a fall in the salt levels in their blood. Severe cramps occur in the calves, the arms and the abdomen. It is now clear that the treatment is to drink fluid containing salt, or milk, and to prevent further cramps occurring by eating salty foods, adding salt to meals, and in the mine drinking fluid containing salt.

At one time miner's nystagmus was a serious cause of disability. This is a twitching of the eyeballs associated with dislike of bright lights, which may appear to be spinning. Other features are giddiness or headache; but sometimes the sufferer has no symptoms at all. Giddiness is the most incapacitating feature and miners with this or other severe symptoms need to be taken away from work underground and from that involving machinery. The disease, which constitutes grounds for compensation under the Workmen's Compensation Act, is caused by prolonged working in poor light, and may take ten to twenty-five years to develop. Better lighting in coal-mines, including whitewashing a number of specified places in the pits, has greatly reduced the incidence of nystagmus, so much so that one distinguished neurologist working in South Wales has stated that he has not seen a new case for twenty years.

Even apart from these occupational risks, however, there is some evidence that miners' health is worse than that of the rest of the community. A joint survey by the Royal College of General Practitioners and the Registrar General found that miners' consultation rates for over half the common illnesses were between two and five times the average for the country as a whole. It seems likely that miners' health and that of other heavy industrial populations is getting worse in relation to the rest of the country, particularly in South Wales. In several recent reports Dr Julian Tudor Hart, a general practitioner in a mining village in South Wales, has shown that not only have miners' wives a higher mortality rate than those of other workers (SMR of 129 in 1959–63), but that the infant mortality – which is probably a better measure of community health – also shows the same discrepancy (SMR of 169 in 1959–63). Unfortunately no data on either of these aspects were given in the Registrar General's most recent *Supplement on Occupational Mortality*, but Dr Tudor Hart has shown from an analysis of his own practice how much serious illness remains in coal-mining communities: of men aged thirty-five to fifty-four and fifty-five to sixty-four, 25 per cent and 61 per cent respectively were disabled. Nevertheless, only 14 per cent of all these men were registered as disabled, probably because this prolongs the time spent in obtaining another job. This means that almost certainly official statistics underestimate the true amount of disability in the community.

Other surveys have confirmed that the consultation rate in general practice for miners is greater than expectation – in South Wales 6·4 consultations per patient per year in mining areas, compared with 4·9 for urban residential and 5·4 for all practices studied. In a national survey the consultation rate for miners for all causes was 124 per cent of the national average, that for bronchitis being 210 per cent and for arthritis and rheumatism 309 per cent. There is much evidence, moreover, to indicate that these high consultation rates are associated with real illness.

HAZARDS AT SEA

Measured by the rates per man of injuries and death, the most dangerous occupation in Britain at present is work offshore in the oil exploration industry. Oil-rig workers have an annual fatality rate of 2–3 per 1,000 – ten times the rate for coal-mining and fifty times that in factories in general. Even more hazardous is the job of deep-sea diving in the North Sea, where the combination of great depths, harsh weather and fast tides creates the worst conditions in the world for this type of work. The current fatality rate is ten per 1,000 even with recent improvements in the training standards of the divers and their medical care.

Despite its replacement by diving as the most hazardous occupation in Britain, trawler-fishing remains highly dangerous. The industry is not large: 7,500 men work through the year to provide 65 per cent of the fish we eat. The number of men killed and injured per year has sometimes been as high as 3,000. In one year when not a single ship capsized the death rate of trawlermen was found to be twice that of fishermen as a whole. The first to produce these figures were Dr Samuel Moore, now area medical officer at York, and Professor Richard Schilling of the London School of Hygiene and Tropical Medicine. Besides spending three weeks on a trawler himself, Dr Moore collected details of all the illnesses, accidents and deaths in trawlermen sailing from Grimsby in 1963 – a difficult and lengthy job when it is remembered that they may have been treated by no fewer than six different agencies, at home or overseas. His search through ships' logbooks and medical records meant that for the first time two really vital pieces of information became available: the number of men sailing from Grimsby that year, and how many days they sailed for. Using them, Dr Moore calculated the rates for accidents, illnesses and death, and hence was able to compare them with the rates for other occupations.

Professor Schilling also became aware of the very high accident rate among trawlermen while he was spending six days at sea investigating a skin disease of fishermen called 'Dogger Bank itch' (p. 152). He found that the death rate from accidents given in the Registrar General's Report did not usually include deaths at sea, which were recorded separately by the Registrar General of Shipping and Seamen. He found that the SMR for accidents at work was 1,726 and that mortality from some other causes was considerably higher than in the general population, particularly high blood pressure and lung and stomach cancer.

Among the total of 2,460 men sailing in 1963 studied by Dr Moore there were 693 injuries and 116 illnesses; of the injuries, 201 were due to falls and slips; 101 to trapping by the gear; ninety-nine to blows and injuries from falling objects; and thirty-four to being knocked down by waves. Half the injuries involved the arms, and a fifth the legs – especially the knee. A total of 143 men had to be put ashore, almost twice as many on account of injury as of illness. Eight men had died from natural causes and six from accidents, giving a death rate from accidents of 2·4 per 1,000.

Most of the injuries suffered by the seamen were caused by falls or blows from the fishing tackle. The trawling gear of a side-trawler weighs ten tons and has to be man-handled several times each shift. The deck is usually covered in blood and slime from the gutting of the fish, and the motion of these relatively small vessels in the mountainous seas is violent and irregular, which gives rise to falls and slips. Trawlermen also get puncture wounds of the skin from wire hawsers and fish bones, and over four out of five of these wounds go septic under the conditions at sea. In the year studied by Dr Moore over 1,000 man-days were lost from infected wounds.

Professor Schilling showed that fatal accidents were commoner in the distant-water fleet than in fishing boats operating in near and middle waters; in side-trawlers compared with the newer stern-trawlers; and in skippers and mates – particularly the latter, who has the most dangerous job of all the deck crew. Between 1957 and 1966 no fewer than ninety trawlers were totally lost or involved in serious accidents, principally owing to negligent navigation or fires together with explosions (which accounted for forty-seven and eighteen instances, respectively). Four vessels were lost in this period during exceptionally severe weather, mainly because of icing of the trawler's superstructure, in conditions of low temperature and strong winds. This made the boat unstable and led it eventually to capsize.

Two other factors which contributed to this high accident rate are physical exhaustion and lack of sleep among the trawlermen, because under the bonus system of payment they have to work excessively long hours. In a near-water trawler Professor Schilling estimated that the deck crew had about six hours' broken rest in twenty-four; this might mean that the men worked 180 hours in ten days of active fishing. Moreover, the men, who spent a relatively short time ashore, might return to their work as tired as when they entered port. 'In a crew which had fished continuously for five days and nights, I became aware of the ashen-grey pallor of their faces, their slower movements, irritability and chain smoking, which reminded me of what I saw among soldiers during the retreat to Dunkirk in 1940,' Professor Schilling commented. The government Committee of Inquiry into Trawler Safety, which was set up after three distant-water Hull trawlers had sunk in 1968 with the loss of fifty-eight men, and on which Professor Schilling served, recommended modest reductions in working hours during fishing and longer periods of shore leave, though these are not yet statutory provisions for the trawling industry. Another way fatigue could be cut down would be to improve the design of the trawlers themselves and their equipment.

Both surveys showed that many men were clearly unfit to be at sea, though at present there is no law to prevent a man with serious heart disease or stomach ulcers from signing on. These problems would be solved by improving the hours and conditions of work, together with a medical examination before entry as well as regular check-ups afterwards. Other things needed are a permanent hospital ship (as provided for the Dutch and German trawlermen) together with refresher courses in first aid and accident prevention for the ships' officers, and improving safety by providing life-lines and non-slip mats, and guarding machinery – all measures which would be compulsory for similar work ashore. Moreover, an accurate weather service would enable the trawlers to avoid conditions liable to lead to severe icing problems.

Probably something like a fifth of fishermen develop occupational skin diseases, and are off sick from this cause for roughly twice as many days as shore workers. These diseases include salt-water boils (septic spots that heal badly because of the effect of sea-water and chafing of the skin), dermatitis due to oil, eczema around the wrists caused by chafing from the cuffs of the waterproof jacket, and Dogger Bank itch. The last, which is particularly prevalent among Lowestoft fishermen, is due to an allergy to the sea-chervil, *Alcyonidium gelatinosum*, a seaweed-like organism which is caught with the fish, and is often commonest in the best fishing grounds. Affected fishermen – who are always trawlermen, since the organism lies on the sea bed and is not caught in drift-nets – develop blistering and rashes on the hands, arms, face and legs, but the rash subsides once the man returns to port. Quite possibly the development of this rash could be prevented by better protective clothing, including gloves, and prototypes are now being tested in use.

INDUSTRIAL ACCIDENTS

Accidents are by far the greatest hazard in industry. Although the annual total has now fallen to about 600 from the 1,000 deaths or more which were occurring only a few years ago, half a million people are still injured in accidents and together with industrial diseases these mean a loss of 19 million working days a year. Most likely even this seriously underestimates the true state of affairs, since, though all accidents causing disability for over three days should be reported by law, probably a quarter of those in the manufacturing industry and half of those in the construction industry are never reported.

The death rate from accidents for the construction industry is five times that in manufacturing industry (in 1972, 20·2 and 3·9 per 100,000 employed, respectively), though the serious-injury rates are less divergent (800 and 580 per 100,000). Even so, whereas the death rate is falling in manufacturing industry, it is not in the construction industry. The Registrar General's *Occupational Mortality Tables* pinpoint the main risks: the SMR for accidents for bricklayers is 72; for plasterers, 55; builders' clerks of works, 80; construction workers not classified, 194; painters and decorators, 116; crane and hoist operators, 225; operators of earth-moving and other construction machinery, 397; and labourers and unskilled workers in building and contracting, 163.

All these figures correspond with the known fatal risks. Falls result in more deaths than any other cause, particularly from unprotected heights, ladders and scaffolding. Accidents associated with transport are the next commonest cause: men on construction sites may be run over, brakes on dumper trucks may fail or their drivers overestimate their capabilities. Falls of ground killed a total of 159 men in a ten-year period, twenty-one of them in 1972. Unless they are supported, trenches may collapse when dug in any type of soil, wet or dry, of a depth between five and twenty feet. Finally, other important causes of death include accidents with lifting equipment, electrocution (sometimes from near-by or overhead power lines), and falls of other materials such as timber or rubble.

As in the manufacturing industry, the prime responsibility for health and safety in the construction industry rests with management, with prevention as the keynote. Many accidents happen through neglect of long-known important precautions – of fencing off heights, shoring up trenches, constructing scaffolding with the right ties and braces. Voluntary bodies such as the Royal Society for the Prevention of Accidents play an important part in producing safety propaganda, while the official role of HM Chief Inspector of Factories includes monitoring accidents, instituting warnings of prosecutions where safety precautions have been ignored (in 1972 no fewer than a quarter of these referred to the construction industry), advising on safety in all its aspects (which includes a permanent display at the Industrial Health and Safety Centre, in London), and putting across these tasks to the workers and public alike.

Ten manufacturing industries showed a particularly high incidence of fatal accidents in 1972, with iron and steel, coke ovens and manufactured fuel, and shipbuilding occupying the three top places. As in the construction industry, falls of workers were the commonest cause, especially from heights, followed by accident involving non-rail transport (in other words, the movement of vehicles in factories), machinery or falls of material all in second place. In his 1972 report the Inspector of Factories said that in only 15 per cent of cases were the events unforeseen or unassessable. The remainder of the fatal accidents might have been prevented by reasonably practicable precautions taken by the management only, the deceased worker only, or both jointly in roughly the same numbers; fellow workers played a lesser part.

Other important types of accidents include fire and explosions, which may occur when liquid oxygen or other gases, petroleum or dusts (including flour) are involved. In 1972 these caused just over 900 injuries, thirteen of them fatal. The recent growth in the use of cellular (foam) plastic in the furniture, motorcar and clothing trades has been accompanied by several serious fires – these foam plastics are highly inflammable.

INDUSTRIAL POISONING

Lead continues to be widely used throughout industry, but it is not now a serious cause of ill-health and there has been only one death from lead poisoning in the last twenty years (compared with 125 deaths in 1900). Technical developments have reduced the amount of lead in paints, though it has been used in newer processes, such as the plastics industry. Much recent publicity has concerned the risks of pollution to the general public (p. 188), but there is still a hard core of notifications of poisoning – a total of eighty-two in 1972 compared with almost 4,000 in 1900. Of these fifteen arose from smelting of metals, fifteen in accumulator works and twenty-five from other works. Special attention still needs to be paid to the first two of these, but there seems little doubt that particular attention to cleanliness (such as swilling down yards and walkways), protective clothing and installing new exhaust ventilation should cut down these figures even further. Another industry where exhaust ventilation may be difficult and the worker closely exposed to lead fumes is ship-breaking, where they arise from burning steel painted with lead paints. Some protection may be obtained from wearing positive-pressure welding visors, but examining the workers and monitoring their blood-lead levels also have important roles.

Lead poisoning seen today is usually much milder than the illness described in the textbooks (p. 197). Special tests have suggested that lead may be having subtle effects on the body of a lead worker who is apparently completely healthy: nerve impulses may take longer to pass down nerve fibres than usual, while the concentration of enzymes in the red blood cells may be reduced.

All this has led to a change of emphasis – in particular to getting away from the concept of lead poisoning to that of lead absorption. This entails measuring the lead levels in the blood and urine as well as those of two other substances in the latter, and enables the condition to be assigned to four categories of lead absorption: normal, acceptable, excessive and dangerous – corresponding to blood-lead levels of 40, 40–80, 80–120 and over 120 mg./100 ml. respectively. Men who are found to have a value of over 80 mg./100 ml. should be closely supervised and taken away from work if they show any tendency to become anaemic. At a level of over 120 mg./100 ml. suspension from work should become automatic. Even the classification based on blood-lead levels (which was produced by an international group of distinguished medical men and scientists) may have

to be revised in the light of the findings of future research –
in particular, the sharp cut-off point of 80 mg./100 ml. may
be an oversimplification – and there remains the difficulty of
measuring lead in the laboratory, which unless meticulously
done may be subject to an error of 30 per cent. Even so, the
need for constant vigilance was spelt out by a large-scale
outbreak of lead poisoning at the Rio Tinto Zinc smelter at
Avonmouth between 1968 and 1971. As the official inquiry
showed, this process was a relatively new one and there were
numerous breakdowns of machinery and spillages. Lead
levels in air rose to 45 mg./cu.m., over 200 times the accepted threshold limit value. Blood levels of up to 220
mg./100 ml. were recorded in spillage cleaners and up to
354 mg./100 ml. in men admitted to hospital, though none
of these suffered any serious or lasting illness. This situation
seems to have arisen because the advanced process presented
great difficulties of hygiene control – despite precautions and
close medical supervision – and it gave rise to what the
official report subsequently described as a 'crisis of
confidence' in the workers at the smelter. The most intrac-
table problem was that of dust control, but following the
report great advances were made in this (with respirators
being used in difficult cases) and the Inspector of Factories
reported no case of reportable lead poisoning up to the end
of 1972 from April of that year, the time the smelter re-
opened.

OCCUPATIONAL CANCER

In 1972 the Inspector of Factories recorded a total of thirty-
six cases of skin cancer – twenty-three due to pitch and tar,
and the remainder to mineral oil. Tumours due to tar and
soot were the first type of occupational cancer to be recognized, when in 1775 Percivall Pott described tumours of the
scrotum arising in chimney-sweeps. In the latter part of the
nineteenth century doctors also recognized tumours of
the exposed parts of the skin in those handling tar, pitch and

shale oil – as in gas-workers producing the first two substances, shale-oil refinery workers, creosoters and road
workers. Shale oil was found to be responsible for mule-spin-
ner's cancer – cancer of the scrotum, limbs or face occurring
in some cotton workers whose clothes or skin became contaminated with lubricating oil thrown off by the spindles of
the machinery.

The cotton industry itself introduced preventive measures
against this risk – protective clothing, works shower baths
and regular six-monthly medical inspection – and these were
reinforced by legislation in 1953, whch made compulsory
the use of white oil, a harmless lubricating substance. Nevertheless, the occupational hazard from mineral oils is still present today – mainly in engineering workers, particularly
tool-setters engaged in manufacturing nuts and bolts, and
those in the jute industry, where jute is softened before it is
woven into cloth by an emulsion of oil and water. These risks
have been recognized only comparatively recently and the
true incidence of this type of cancer is still not known (certainly in relation to occupation), but probably both would be
reduced by the same precautions taken in the cotton-spin-
ning industry.

Another occupational tumour, whose risk has not greatly
diminished, is that of the bladder, or occasionally of other
urinary passages such as the ureter and the collecting area of
the kidney. This usually starts as a benign growth of the
lining of the passages, which becomes malignant later if not
treated. Occupational urinary cancer was first discovered in
the aniline dyestuffs industry in Germany in 1895, thirty
years after the manufacturing process had been introduced,
when three out of a total of forty-five workers making
magenta were found to have bladder cancer. Research
showed much later that the responsible agent was not aniline itself but the chemicals naphthylamine and ben-
zidine, and we now know that seven such substances may
produce this type of cancer. In Britain these dyes were not
manufactured until after the First World War, and the first

cases of occupational bladder tumours were described in 1929.

Other manufacturing processes using these chemicals also started at that time, in particular antoxidants containing naphthylamine were widely used to prevent rubber perishing in the manufacture of rubber tyres, tubes and cables. There was a delay in recognizing the risks, for two main reasons. Firstly, the disease may have a very long latent period – up to forty years from exposure, with an average of eighteen years. Often by the time a man develops the tumour he has moved to another job and the connection between the two goes unrecognized, particularly since cancer of the bladder is fairly common (killing about 4,000 people a year in Britain). When screening methods were introduced, by examining the urine under the microscope for blood cells and tumour cells, it was estimated that 50,000 people might have been at risk at some time. But of the 43,000 contacted, only 2,500 came forward to have this simple examination. Hence an accurate assessment of the risk is difficult, though individual small-scale studies have provided valuable evidence: of 667 workers exposed in Manchester, 123 were found to have developed bladder tumours, and the incidence in those exposed for thirty years or over was 71 per cent. Extrapolating from these findings, there were probably between 400 and 450 cases of bladder tumours among men employed in the rubber industry, some of whom had left it. The second reason was that research in animals was lengthy and difficult, since only dogs develop tumours after being given these substances.

Other, smaller groups of workers might be exposed, either to the substances themselves or to traces of them contaminating otherwise harmless materials. There is a risk to textile printers who have used these substances in dyeing cloth; to the laboratory workers who have used them in various tests; and to rat-catchers who have used rodenticides containing them as impurities; to retort-house workers in the gas industry; and possibly also to hand-tailors and hairdressers. Tumours of the urinary passages have become commoner this century, partly because of smoking (p. 248) and partly due to occupational exposure. Though we have no precise figures, possibly 20 per cent of all bladder tumours have an occupational origin.

The manufacture of naphthylamine for treating rubber was abandoned in 1949, as soon as the risks became known. Industrial benefit for conditions due to these substances became payable in 1967, while their import was prohibited two years later. So far it has proved impossible to develop alternative methods of making the dyes, but these are now manufactured under closely controlled conditions, with regular medical supervision of the workers.

OCCUPATIONAL DERMATITIS

Many people tend to develop skin irritation and a mild rash when they start working in a new industrial process, but in most cases these disappear within a few weeks because the skin has become 'hardened', either by actual physical toughening or by developing some kind of immunity. Even so, some workers develop permanent dermatitis which compels them to take time off work; this is more likely in men than in women, in those who have a greasy complexion and in those over fifty. There are two main causes of occupational dermatitis: the primary irritants and the sensitizers. The primary irritants which cause most trouble include substances removing greases from the skin (such as alkalis, soap, alcohol and water), friction and sweating. A wide range of sensitizing agents may produce an allergic rash in a sensitive person, but only a small proportion of the whole working population will react in this way. They include various plants and woods, coal-tar products, explosives, fertilizers, photographic chemicals, dyes, antibiotics and plasticizers.

It is often difficult to diagnose occupational dermatitis, and in particular to distinguish it from ordinary eczema: the condition has to start at work; the site of onset and the distribution of the rash need to be the places most exposed to the agent; the precise cause needs to be identified and other workers as well as the patient have to appear affected. Even so, even with these criteria there are often difficulties: less than 20 per cent of cases of eczema of the hand turn out to be of industrial origin.

If a worker can avoid contact with the particular sensitizer which provokes his dermatitis – by changing his method of working or wearing protective appliances such as gloves – the outlook is good. It is less good, however, for a person whose skin has broken down as a result of exposure to primary irritants – though with education, supervision and protection it is often possible for a man to keep working at his original job without further difficulty.

OTHER INDUSTRIAL DISEASES

Although several other diseases are notifiable under the Factories Act, only four others are mentioned with any regularity in the Inspector's report: cadmium poisoning, aniline poisoning, compressed-air illness and chrome ulceration. Cadmium poisoning occurs when men are exposed to the metal fume, usually in cutting or welding in an enclosed place metal plated with cadmium to prevent corrosion. Most often the symptoms come on a short time after exposure and include a feeling of being off-colour, shivering, sweating, cough and shortness of breath. This last reflects involvement of the lungs and may become serious, sometimes resulting in death. Occasionally workers may be poisoned by long-term exposure to cadmium, affecting either the lungs or sometimes the kidneys.

There were seven cases of cadmium poisoning in 1972, none of them fatal. In the same year there were fifteen cases of aniline poisoning, with no fatalities. Used extensively in the dye, chemical and explosives industry, aniline is readily absorbed through the skin and alters the haemoglobin in the red blood cells so that the blood may turn brown while the person may become a bluish-grey colour – particularly the lips, tongue, ears and nose. Death is possible though now unusual. Prolonged mild poisoning may occur, with weakness, giddiness and shortness of breath. Aniline poisoning may be prevented by manufacturing and using it and its derivatives in closed systems and placing particular emphasis on speedy removal of splashed clothing.

There was a total of 130 cases of chrome ulceration in 1972, sixty-seven in the manufacture of bichromates, sixty-one in chromium plating, and two in other industries. Ulcers most commonly occur on the fingers, hands or nose – where they may perforate the membrane that separates the two sides of the nose (and make the man whistle in his sleep). On the hands these ulcers usually develop after six months of working with chromium; the itching they produce may keep the sufferer awake at night, but they tend to heal. The person whose nasal septum is perforated usually experiences no trouble from it. These ulcers are prevented by exhaust ventilation in chromium-plating works and by the use of rubber gloves. Regular medical inspection of the workers is required by statute to see if they have developed chrome ulcers, but the value of this has been questioned.

In a few cases exposure to chromium fumes may cause asthma. More serious is the association between the refining of chromium ore and lung cancer, which at one time affected between 20 and 25 per cent of the employees involved. A similar risk existed in the refining of nickel ore, though this does not now take place in Britain.

Serious decompression illness, as recorded in the Inspector of Factories' annual reports of the last few years, has ranged from fifty-one cases including one death to none at all. This disease occurs in workers constructing tunnels and using compressed-air caissons at pressures over 18 lb./sq. in. Symptoms occur in those who undergo decompression too fast, in divers who surface too rapidly, and in airmen who ascend too high in unpressurized air. During compression before and during work in these circumstances gas (almost entirely nitrogen) is forced from the bloodstream into the tissues. If the person is brought back to normal pressure quickly, nitrogen bubbles are formed in the tissues.

Decompression occurs in two main forms. The first includes the 'niggles' (mild pains in the arms and legs or in the major joints); the 'bends' (more severe pains in these joints); and the 'itches' (discoloration of the skin and irritation). The second type is much more serious and includes severe sickness; 'the staggers' (with giddiness, tingling, and numbness and weakness of the limbs); 'the chokes' (shortness of breath, severe headache and symptoms of heart involvement); and even death. Both types must be treated by recompressing the sufferer in a compression chamber and then slowly decompressing him to allow the tissues to expel the nitrogen without forming any bubbles. Decompression in stages by halving the pressure at each stage and prolonging the final ones is always safe, but boring for the men undergoing it, who are tempted to cut the last stages short. For this reason, continual research is going on into different schedules and methods for compression and decompression.

Divers working deep beneath the North Sea on oil pipelines must acclimatize themselves to very high pressures, and when using 'saturation' methods a diver may remain under pressure for as long as a month, spending his rest periods in a pressure chamber on the rig or the supply ship. In these circumstances a medical emergency such as a perforated stomach ulcer can present serious problems, since the decompression procedure cannot be speeded up: the initial treatment may need to be given inside the chamber.

Another risk run by compressed-air workers is caisson bone disease. In this condition small areas of bone are destroyed, and when this occurs near a joint it may eventually cause arthritis. Possibly as many as a fifth of people working at high pressures have these changes in their bones – about half with lesions near the joints. There seems to be little link between the development of caisson bone disease and the occurrence of the bends or more serious illness or the number of exposures to working in compressed air. But X-ray surveys of the bones of workers in caissons are now usually done routinely, while episodes of serious bends have to be notified to the Inspector of Factories, including the proportion of cases needing treatment by recompression. If the latter rises above 2 per cent of all compressions then an inquiry is initiated.

ANTHRAX

No cases of anthrax were notified in 1972 or 1971, but there were four cases in 1969 (one of them fatal), and a total of forty-six cases in that and the preceding few years. Anthrax is a serious infection, usually of the skin, but sometimes of the lungs or bloodstream, caused by a bacterium called *Bacillus anthracis*. Primarily it infects cattle, the human disease being acquired from spores of the germ present in hides, fleeces, bones or bone meal, and horn. This mode of transmission gave rise to the term 'wool-sorter's disease', after the lung condition caused by inhaling spores released from fleeces, but most cases affect the skin and many are acquired from infected bone meal. The infection usually starts as a small pimple at the point of contact of the skin with the infected hide or bone meal. If untreated, this rapidly becomes larger with a black centre and considerable swelling, though it may heal itself. Infection of the lung is usually as a virulent pneumonia, while that of the bloodstream is a serious generalized illness with high temperature and sweating; fortunately the disease usually clears up quickly with antibiotic treatment, such as penicillin.

Brushes made from goat hair have to be sterilized under an Act of Parliament, at the Government Wool Disinfecting Station. Although some other hides and fleeces or consignments of bones or bone meal are sterilized when they are imported into this country, legally they do not have to be, and workers in high-risk industries are now encouraged to be vaccinated against it. They are also provided with cards stating their occupational risk to show to their doctors, so that an early diagnosis may be made.

DUST DISEASES

Besides coal-workers' pneumoconiosis (see pp. 143–6) three types of serious dust disease are still encountered in industry: silicosis, asbestosis and allergic lung diseases. Silicosis is a disease of the lungs due to inhalation of dust containing uncombined silica. This provokes the formation of scar tissues throughout the lungs, and often is complicated by the development of tuberculosis and large aggregated masses of scar tissue. The duration of exposure to silica before the condition appears varies from six months to sixty years, but is said to average five years. Symptoms vary according to the severity of the changes in the lung – from mild shortness of breath to severe heart failure – and may be complicated by tuberculosis.

Silicon forms about a quarter of the earth's crust, so that not surprisingly exposure to the dust was a common risk before the link between dust and disease was discovered. Particularly at risk were quarrymen and stonemasons working with sandstone or granite; pottery workers; tin, coal and graphite miners working in seams where silica was present; slate-quarrying; metal-grinding and casting; and sand-blasting. The risks from all of these have been reduced by the use of substitutes where possible, as in the pottery industry, or by dust suppression – including cutting rock wet, exhaust ventilation and individual respirators. By law all deaths from notifiable industrial diseases have to be reported to the coroner and in 1971 just over 100 deaths were registered in Britain from pneumoconiosis linked with industries. This compares with just over 1,000 deaths mentioning coal-miners' pneumoconiosis, but whereas many new cases of the latter are still occurring, most cases of silicosis seen now have arisen as a result of exposure some years before.

Asbestosis is another type of scarring of the lungs due to the inhalation of asbestos fibres, but it differs from silicosis in several ways. In asbestosis concomitant tuberculosis is rarer, but serious illness is commoner as scarring of the lung progresses more rapidly. Men with asbestosis are also particularly liable to develop cancer of the lung: the risk has been put at between 10 and 50 per cent by various authorities. This risk, however, is present only in smokers so that tobacco seems to act synergistically with asbestos in producing the condition.

Asbestosis was first recognized in 1930 and the regulations introduced three years later to enforce dust suppression seem to have been very effective; certainly the incidence of asbestosis has fallen. Even so, the world production of asbestos has shot up and this valuable and often indispensable material is said to be used now in over 1,000 separate ways – in lagging pipes, constructional work and brake linings in cars. This means that workers outside asbestos mines or factories may be exposed to asbestos dust; for example, shipwrights engaged in lagging pipes or lining cabins with insulation board, as well as their mates doing tasks not involving asbestos but working alongside them and being exposed to the dust. An estimated total of at least 20,000 workers in Britain may be exposed to some form of asbestos. But whereas asbestosis has not occurred very frequently in these workers – because it seems to be due to the inhalation of massive amounts of dust – other more subtle effects have now been recognized. The first is the presence of 'plaques' – small fibrous thickenings on the pleura (the membrane lining the surface of the lung), which have been found in between 5 and 33 per cent of shipworkers, depending on their job, and in about 18 per cent of joiners in building work. The second effect was recognized only in 1960 and is a malignant tumour of the pleura called mesothelioma. Some of these tumours have been observed to develop from pleural plaques.

Mesotheliomas used to be regarded as very rare, but they are now diagnosed not infrequently and at least 80 per cent of them occur in people with some exposure to asbestos. Indeed, of the 413 people with mesothelioma seen in 1967–8, at least two thirds had been engaged in manufacturing asbestos products or using asbestos for insulation work. Similar tumours of the membrane lining the abdominal cavity or of the intestines are occasionally seen in people with similar occupational exposure to asbestos. Characteristically these tumours develop after a long period of exposure (forty-three years on average), but exposure need be neither heavy nor prolonged.

All these new risks were recognized in regulations introduced in 1969, which insist on exhaust ventilation or, if this is impossible, on the use of protective clothing and protective breathing equipment. Since the risk of mesothelioma is particularly great with blue asbestos (crocidolite), compared with the white or brown varieties (chrysotile and amosite, respectively) the district inspector of factories has to be notified of any process in which the first is being used.

Finally, the question arises whether the general population is at any risk from inhaling asbestos. The lungs of many town dwellers contain a few asbestos bodies, and at least two women are known to have developed asbestosis through holding sheet asbestos for their husbands, one of whom was building a bungalow and the other a rabbit hutch. But in general the risk is probably very low for ordinary exposure.

FARMER'S LUNG

Lung disease may also result from the inhalation of vegetable dusts, usually from allergy to mould contained in them. This results in illness – with fever, breathlessness and muscle pains – often followed by asthma a few hours later. 'Farmer's lung' occurs in farmworkers exposed to mouldy hay (as during threshing) because they have developed an allergy to the fungus *Micropolyspora faeni* contained in it. Very occasionally if the farmer has a number of these attacks he may develop scarring of the lung tissue, bronchitis and breathlessness. The same type of condition is seen in workers handling bagasse (bagassosis), the cellulose fibre of sugar-cane imported into this country for manufacture into hardboard. In this case the condition is due to allergy to other types of fungi, including *Aspergillus fumigatus*.

Exposure to cotton contaminated with a fungus may produce a similar illness to farmer's lung, but there is a much commoner lung disease in workers in the cotton industry whose cause is still not known. This illness, called byssinosis, occurs in some form in about one fifth of the workers, and is commoner in those who smoke. In its early stages it consists of tightness in the chest and fever, usually occurring on return to work after the week-end (called 'Monday fever'). Usually a person has worked in the industry for about ten years before he develops byssinosis and if he leaves it the condition subsides. If he stays, however, the disease may progress into disabling attacks of asthma or bronchitis, and possibly eventually into crippling breathlessness. Though there has been considerable progress in reducing the amount of dust in the cotton industry and the incidence of disabling byssinosis is decreasing, deaths are still being notified from this cause, and in 1971 totalled twenty-one.

OTHER OCCUPATIONAL HAZARDS

The number of other occupational hazards is legion, and even a few lines on each could occupy a whole book. But in most cases both the causes and the remedies have been known for some time. For example, effective personal ear-muffs will protect against the occupational deafness which occurs in cotton workers and boilermakers (the problem of noise is discussed under pollution: p. 198). Safe handling procedures will eliminate the risk of infections acquired in bacteriological laboratory workers or in animal-handlers. And keeping scrupulously to the recommended code of practice for the use of radioactive materials and X-ray machines (which are increasingly employed in industry and on construction sites) should prevent radiation injuries, which in 1972 still totalled sixty-three – one of them involving severe injury to a radiographer's hand, caused by inadequately protected equipment. Even workers in nuclear power stations should run no risk of radiation illness if the safety procedures are followed; the real hazard comes when an accident occurs, as happened at Windscale, Cumberland, in 1957. Treatment of acute radiation injury has been much improved in recent years, however, so that short of a major explosion occurring the new generation of nuclear power stations should not present a health hazard either to workers or to the public. The risk of explosion is a contentious matter: despite reassuring statements from the authorities most of us would prefer not to have a potential nuclear bomb within range of our homes.

Even so, new hazards may arise from new processes. Biological washing powders were mentioned at the beginning of this chapter; another danger was also recognized only a few years ago and arose out of the rapidly increasing popularity of isocyanates or polyurethanes – which in some workers produces a pattern of lung disease similar to farmer's lung or byssinosis: at first asthma, followed by permanent lung damage. These are widely used in upholstery, car seats, packaging materials and paints. Once manufactured, these compounds are completely harmless, and with production running at 10,000 tons a year in Britain they are found in almost every home.

During the manufacturing process, however, the isocyanate is mixed with resin. The resulting chemical reaction generates heat, which releases the dangerous compound tolylene diisocyanate (TID) into the surrounding air.

Prolonged exposure to TID in concentrations above 0·1 p.p.m. (parts per million) irritates the eyes, throat and lungs; and some workers have developed a sensitivity reaction such as asthma to the chemical and have had to change their jobs. Manufacturers usually aim to keep the concentration of TID in the air at less than 0·02 p.p.m. But the latest research shows that even at this level there is a steady, slight deterioration in the workers' lungs, which is faster than in bronchitis (though the rate is still slow).

Again the answer has been to monitor the workers' health and the concentration of TID in the air, reducing the latter by exhaust ventilation or using substitutes where practicable. Another risk was subsequently tackled in the same way when fumes were found to be released in cutting foam slabs. Even so some people still seem to be unaware of the inherent risks of these substances; for example, in his 1972 report the Inspector of Factories stated that they were still being used in the restoration of works of art.

Recognition has yet to be given to the less obvious forms of occupational disease, many of which are preventable. How many typists finish the day with backache because their chairs were not designed for the job? The better industrial designers are fully aware of the new science of ergonomics, which aims to increase efficiency by providing optimum physical working conditions, but as yet many employers prefer to spend money on décor rather than better furniture. Legislation exists defining minimum standards of lighting, space, heating, toilet facilities and so on; but again there are wide variations in the attention paid to these regulations by different employers.

WORKERS' RIGHTS

There is some truth in the charge that unions and indeed workers are more concerned with compensation than with prevention. Only too often there is a conflict between productivity and safety, and it may be possible for a worker paid at piece rates to earn more if he removes the guard from a machine. Again, it is difficult to persuade workers to wear protective clothing or masks to reduce the risks of disease developing twenty or thirty years later. For these reasons the Factories Acts and related legislation lay absolute duties on employees to observe fundamental precautions such as machinery guards, and any worker who sees a breach of the regulations can inform the local factory inspector. If a worker suspects that there is a health hazard in his work but is uncertain of the legal position he can get advice from the local community physician employed by his area health authority. In such cases, however, the local trade union officials will usually be able to advise and conciliate. The same advice applies when a worker has in fact suffered illness as a result of his work: his union is the best arbiter in persuading the employer to find alternative work if it is available.

LOW-MORTALITY-RATE OCCUPATIONS

All the recent Registrar General's analyses of SMR by social class have shown a gradient of mortality according to social class. Between 1959 and 1963 the SMRs for men were: social class I (professional and executive occupations), 76; II (managerial and administrative occupations), 81; III (skilled occupations), 100; IV (partly skilled occupations), 103; and V (unskilled occupations), 143. For classes I and II SMRs have improved since 1930–32, with a particular improvement recently in the rates for middle-aged lawyers, teachers and clergymen. The SMRs for class V have, however, deteriorated considerably – from 111 in 1930–32 to 143 in 1959–63 – though whether this is all real is difficult to say.

The persistently low SMRs of some occupations might suggest that these had no inherent hazards, but this is not always the case. Thus one of our biggest industries, farming, has an SMR of 72 for farmers and farm managers, and of 89 for agricultural labourers. Even so, every year there are about 9,000 accidents and diseases in agriculture reported to the Ministry of Agriculture (certainly an underestimate), of which 120 are fatal. Tractor accidents cause 20 per cent of the injuries and half of the deaths – mostly through over-turning on steep slopes. Falls (from vehicles, ladders, trees and haystacks) cause another 20 per cent of the injuries and almost 30 per cent of the deaths, while animals account for 10 per cent and 6 per cent respectively: every year about seven deaths are caused by animals, five of them from attacks by bulls (the commonest animal to injure farm-workers). Other risks include infections – Weil's disease, anthrax, brucellosis (p. 81), Q fever and tetanus – farmer's lung (p. 166), asphyxiation from carbon dioxide produced in grain silos, and eye injuries from foreign bodies entering the eye. Thus the farm may appear to be a safe place to work, but there are hidden hazards for the unwary.

Chapter 8

DISEASES FROM PETS

FROM time to time a newspaper headline announces: 'Woman dies from parrot disease', and there is a rush of articles warning of health hazards from pet animals. In practice these risks are very small. Over 6 million dogs are licensed in Britain, and there are certainly as many cats and budgerigars; other families keep tropical fish, gerbils or rabbits, and a few have pet monkeys or boa constrictors; but each year the number of serious illnesses due to these animals is limited to a few hundred. The risks, then, are small, and can be reduced to a negligible level by a few sensible hygienic precautions.

DOGS AND CATS

Fortunately for the British, rabies, which is by far the most dangerous illness communicated by animals, has been kept out of the United Kingdom by rigid quarantine laws. Rabies is one of the few human diseases with virtually 100 per cent mortality – there is only one recorded case of a cure – and it is a growing problem in Europe and North America, spreading every year, to affect Scandinavia for the first time for decades. It is transmitted by a bite from an infected, maddened or paralysed animal, and anyone bitten by a dog or cat that could possibly have rabies is recommended to have precautionary vaccination against the disease.

In Britain perhaps the most important disease carried by dogs and cats is toxocariasis. Very few people have heard of the condition – which is not surprising since it is less than twenty-five years since it was first recognized as a human disease.

Dogs and cats carry in their intestines parasitic worms,

toxocara, which may grow up to 5 in. (12·5 cm) long. These worms lay eggs which can infect other dogs, cats and men. When an adult or child swallows toxocara eggs they hatch in the intestines, penetrate the bowel wall, and so reach the bloodstream. The larvae travel in the bloodstream to every part of the body, particularly the lungs and the liver. A child that swallows many toxocara eggs may develop a feverish illness, visceral larva migrans, with a cough and some swelling and tenderness of the liver. Usually this illness subsides without much difficulty: but if the larvae reach the brain or the eye more serious illness may result. Brain infection may lead to epilepsy; larvae which reach the eye may set up a chronic inflammation leading to blindness.

Tests done at the London School of Hygiene suggest that about 2 per cent of the population have been infected with toxocara at some time in their lives – almost certainly in childhood. Serious eye disease from this cause is still a rarity, however. Nevertheless, small children should not be allowed to play in soil which may have been contaminated by excreta from dogs or cats.

A series of tests done by the London School of Hygiene showed that soil in public parks is usually heavily contaminated with toxocara, and children aged one to four – the age at which normal activity includes crawling around flowerbeds – may become infected, but in practice very few do develop symptoms of toxocariasis. Nevertheless public pressure is needed to discourage the current attitude that permits dogs and cats to contaminate any property in a city, public or private.

The life-cycle of the toxocara worm is (like that of many parasites) complicated. When a bitch becomes pregnant larvae migrate to the womb, where they infect the puppies before birth. Puppies are the greatest source of infection, for if they have been infected before birth they pass toxocara eggs in large quantities in their faeces. Since puppies are messy creatures, and since children and puppies often play together there is a high risk of infection. The best defence against this risk is treatment of the puppies at about three weeks to eradicate any infection that may be present. Good pet shops do this before selling a puppy. Infection before birth does not seem to occur with the toxocara that affects cats, and kittens are not so likely to be carriers of the disease. Nevertheless, it is safer to de-worm kittens too.

Toxocariasis should be distinguished from toxoplasmosis, another parasitic disease which may be acquired from contact with cats. Usually the disease is trivial: and laboratory tests show that about one adult in three has been infected at some time. However, if a pregnant woman becomes infected the parasites may pass to the unborn child, where they can cause serious damage to the brain and other organs. About one in every 30,000 babies is born with congenital toxoplasmosis: the condition responds to drug treatment if it is recognized at birth, but this cannot cure the damage already done.

Catscratch fever is said to be the most common disease that man can catch from cats. Within ten to twenty days of an apparently trivial scratch the person develops swollen, tender lymph nodes that drain the area of the scratch — usually the nodes at the elbow or in the armpit. The scratch wound itself may become obviously inflamed, and other symptoms may include fever, loss of appetite and a general feeling of being off colour. Sometimes the swollen glands settle down within a week or two; on other occasions a liquid discharge may appear from the swollen glands.

The disease is unpleasant and worrying, since it may be difficult in the early stage for it to be distinguished from more serious conditions such as Hodgkin's disease. As yet the causative agent (which is presumably a virus) has not been identified, nor is there any specific treatment, but antibiotics seem to shorten the disease and reduce its severity.

Many other parasites may be acquired from dogs, including tapeworms or their cystic forms, though this is rare in Britain; dog fleas and lice may infest man, but they rarely cause serious trouble. Man may also be infected with the fungus of mange or ringworm and the spirochaetes of lepto-spirosis. Leptospirosis (Weil's disease) is common in rats and is transmitted to man by contact with water contaminated with rat urine. It is therefore an occupational hazard for sewer workers and a risk for anyone falling into a canal or river who swallows any amount of water. The disease causes jaundice and a high fever and may be dangerous, but it may sometimes be cured by antibiotic treatment. These infections, however, are sufficient rarities to be reported in medical journals should they occur. Allergy to fur and hairs of cats and dogs is a not uncommon cause of asthma, and, as in other forms of allergic asthma, diagnosis and treatment depend on someone spotting the association.

BIRDS

There are two important diseases transmitted from birds to man: psittacosis (parrot fever) and bird-fancier's lung.

Psittacosis is caused by bedsoniae, micro-organisms midway in size between viruses and bacteria. It is so called because it is a disease of the psittacine or parrot family: it affects at least seventy different types of bird, including budgerigars, cockatoos and macaws; pigeons and doves; domestic poultry; seagulls; and many types of finch, including canaries.

Most birds infected with psittacosis have no features of the illness and the disease is generally low-grade. This probably explains the low infectivity of the disease for man. It is rare for human infection to occur even among men or women in daily contact with birds. Sometimes, however, an apparently healthy bird can infect many people – as on one occasion when twelve actors caught psittacosis from a stage parrot. Possibly the strains of bedsoniae that affect parrots and turkeys are more virulent than the others; certainly psittacosis is a recognized hazard among workers who handle turkey carcases.

In practice, though psittacosis is a theoretical risk for

anyone who comes into contact with birds, in most serious cases reported in Britain there has been a clear history of prolonged association with a sickly cage-bird, usually a parrot.

Human psittacosis is a feverish illness, with generalized aches and pains and a cough. The main target organ is the lungs, and psittacotic pneumonia may threaten life. Modern treatment with broad-spectrum antibiotics is usually curative if the condition is diagnosed reasonably early: one series of 550 cases included only three deaths. Anyway, only a handful of serious cases have been reported in Britain since the prohibition on the importation of birds was lifted in 1966.

Allergy to birds' feathers or eggs is quite common among families who keep cage-birds or who look after domestic fowls. Any of the typical forms of allergic response may be found – asthma, urticaria (raised red blotches on the skin), or sneezing and watering of the eyes. In such cases skin tests may be used to confirm the hypersensitivity, and the standard treatment is then given – either a course of desensitizing injections or drug treatment to relieve the symptoms.

Bird-fancier's lung is a more serious form of hypersensitivity, and is usually caused by inhalation of dust from the dried droppings of budgerigars, parrots or pigeons. The hypersensitivity does not cause typical allergic symptoms such as asthma: instead, the internal lining of the lungs becomes thickened where it comes into contact with the inhaled particles of dust.

Symptoms include cough, shortness of breath, episodes of fever, shivering, loss of weight and a general feeling of ill-health. Usually the disease runs a slow course, but acute attacks may come on when a hypersensitive individual cleans out a bird-cage. The only effective treatment (as with the medically similar condition of farmer's lung due to inhalation of dust from mouldy hay; p. 166) consists of protection against further inhalation of dust, either by a change of occupation, getting rid of the birds, or providing the patient with a dust-mask to wear while attending to the birds.

FISH, AMPHIBIANS AND TORTOISES

Few diseases which affect fish have any dangers for man: but there are one or two exceptions. Several cases have been reported in recent years of a form of chronic skin disease found among owners of tropical fish tanks. Characteristically, a trivial cut on the hand fails to heal and after a few weeks small swellings like boils appear around the original lesion. These nodules may extend up the arm as far as the shoulder. The illness is likely to puzzle doctors unless they discover the vital clue – recent disease among tropical fish looked after by the patient.

The bacterium responsible for both the death of the fish and the skin disease in man is a slow-growing relative of the tuberculosis bacillus. *Mycobacterium marinum* is found wherever there is warm water, particularly in heated swimming pools and in tropical fish tanks. It may be brought into a healthy fish tank in water fleas obtained from ponds, and often it persists in a dormant state in cracks in the wall of a swimming bath or an old well. Human infection occurs when someone cleaning an aquarium has a cut or graze on his hand which allows the bacteria to enter. Once recognized, the infection can usually be readily cured by anti-tuberculosis drugs. Even without treatment, however, the human infection usually resolves spontaneously within six to thirty months.

A much more acute illness may be caught from terrapins, the warm-water miniature turtles that have become very popular in recent years. Each year several outbreaks of diarrhoea and vomiting due to infection with salmonellae (bacteria that cause food poisoning; p. 60) have been traced to terrapins. Typically, the disease is spread when children play with the terrapins, since both their excreta and the water in which they are kept are usually heavily infected with these bacteria. Children given terrapins as pets should be warned to wash their hands carefully after handling them or cleaning out the tank. Water from the tank should not be emptied down the kitchen sink, since it may splash onto surfaces used for the preparation of food; nor should the dishes used for feeding terrapins or turtles be washed up with other domestic utensils.

The small, Greek tortoise so often bought as a garden pet is said to be a carrier of salmonellae, but in practice outbreaks of diarrhoea rarely seem to be traced to these animals – so that the risk seems small, especially in the light of the hundreds and thousands of tortoises in Britain.

MONKEYS

No pet is less suitable for the amateur than a monkey. Dr B. Bisseru, in his detailed book on the medical aspects of pets,* states that monkeys

as pets need a lot of attention and are expensive to feed. Every year monkeys are offered to zoos all over Britain by people who, having bought them as pets, find them unmanageable. Monkeys and the larger apes are easily enraged, strong, temperamental, unpredictable and dangerous, and will attack and bite readily. Completely tame and trustworthy monkeys are rare.

Unfortunately, in addition to these hazards monkeys can also carry several serious diseases, and at present no quarantine is imposed when they are imported into Britain. Though rare, monkey B virus is important since it can cause a brain infection that is usually fatal for man but is less serious for monkeys. The disease is recognized as an occupational hazard among laboratory staff working with monkeys, who get the illness by a bite or scratch. Hence laboratory workers, circus staff and other professionals are very circumspect in handling new arrivals from abroad.

* Bisseru, B., *Diseases of Man Acquired from his Pets*, London, Heinemann, 1967.

Marburg disease is another rare disease of monkeys; when it affects man it causes liver damage and interferes with the normal process of blood-clotting. It gets its name from the German city where an outbreak of the disease among laboratory workers caused seven deaths in 1967. Marburg disease shares with B virus the unenviable qualities of high infectivity and lack of any curative treatment. Little is known about how the monkeys get these infections, but they seem to be brought into laboratory animal houses by new arrivals from Africa. In addition to these two unusual conditions monkeys may carry many other viruses, including rabies, and most doctors think that they are quite unsuitable as family pets.

LEUKAEMIA AND PETS

One recurrent medical scare-story that sometimes gets into the popular press is the risk of animals being a source of leukaemia. The basis of this story is the undoubted fact that one form of leukaemia does affect domestic cats and is transmitted by a virus. Surely, the argument runs, there is a possibility that this virus could infect children playing with their pets, and so perhaps be a cause of childhood leukaemia?

It is never easy to disprove a theory of this kind, but as far as is possible it has been done. Doctors in the Oxford University Department of Social Medicine have been studying cancer in childhood for over twenty years. One of the questions always asked of families of children with cancer was the type of pet that had been kept. The results showed that the proportion keeping pets was virtually identical in the families of 243 children with leukaemia, 257 cases of other types of cancer, and 500 controls.

The view taken by cancer experts now seems to be that it is impossible to rule out the chance that an occasional case of childhood leukaemia could have been due to a cat leukaemia virus; but that such transmission plays little part in the causation of human cancers.

Chapter 9

DETERGENTS; COSMETICS AND OTHER VANITIES

DETERGENTS

DETERGENTS have become one of the worst villains in campaigns against pollution, largely as a result of their obvious unsightly effects on rivers and streams, which so often are covered in layers of indestructible foam. They have nearly as bad a reputation among housewives, who blame them for almost any skin disorder affecting the hands.

Detergents can cause two distinct types of skin disorder. Dishpan hands are very common among people who do a lot of hand-washing of clothes and dishes. The redness, cracking and scaling of the skin are not an allergic reaction to a particular detergent: they simply result from repeated damage to the skin. Detergents remove some of the natural protective oils from the skin: repeated immersion in water softens it, and when this is combined with inadequate drying, hanging up washing in cold and windy conditions, and the damage caused by wringing and squeezing washing it is not surprising that the skin becomes chronically inflamed.

Less often the skin suffers a genuine allergic reaction to a constituent of the detergent powder, and an allergic eczema, detergent dermatitis, develops. When this is suspected the diagnosis can be confirmed by a patch test on a non-exposed area of skin such as the back.

Reactions of this kind to detergents have remained relatively rare. When enzyme detergents were first introduced several reports suggested that severe reactions were likely to these new compounds: but large-scale tests by the makers on over 7,000 housewives showed that the enzyme powders were no worse than conventional detergents. There is a risk of allergy among the workers concerned with the manufacture of enzyme detergents who may inhale the enzymes in dust in the factory; but this risk has now been recognized and the necessary safety procedures have been introduced.

Soaps are 'kinder' to the skin than detergents, largely because they are less caustic. Oily toilet soap is intrinsically benign, but there is a risk of allergic reactions to additives such as perfumes and colouring matter. Once again the diagnosis can be confirmed by specific testing – but it has to be suspected first.

HEXACHLORAPHANE

Soaps are available with added germicides or other compounds designed to remove bacteria from the skin. For many years the best-known of these agents was hexachloraphane, a chemical related to carbolic acid, which has a powerful antibacterial action. Unlike phenol, hexachloraphane (spelt 'hexachlorophene' in the USA) is not caustic, and it retains its antibacterial action in the presence of soap, so in the early 1950s it became very popular as an additive to soaps. In Britain and the USA a dilute solution of hexachloraphane was used almost universally in hospitals for bathing newborn infants to prevent them picking up bacterial skin infections; and many surgeons used a proprietary mixture of hexachloraphane, lanolin and a detergent (Phisohex) for washing their hands.

Suddenly in 1971 a bombshell exploded with the publication in the *Lancet* of results of experiments on rats suggesting that brain damage could result from prolonged exposure to hexachloraphane. The brain disorder found in these rats was very similar in appearance to a human disease, spongy degeneration of the brain, that sometimes caused deaths in infants and for which the cause was unknown. Had hexachloraphane been responsible for some of these cases? Certainly tests showed that when newborn babies were bathed with 3 per cent hexachloraphane solutions, appreciable quantities of the chemical could be detected in the bloodstream, and some of a group of newborn monkeys bathed regularly with the solution developed the characteristic spongy degeneration of the brain. All this evidence was suggestive, but it was based on animal experiments and had to be set against the millions of babies who had been bathed – apparently without ill-effect – in hexachloraphane and the convincing evidence that this treatment prevented deaths from bacterial skin infections.

However, the USA Food and Drugs Administration took its usually cautious line and ordered that 3 per cent hexachloraphane should be distributed only by prescription and that all containers should be labelled 'not for routine bathing'. Consumer organizations took up the crusade, and when in late 1972 there were reports from France of deaths of some infants said to be due to excessive use of 6 per cent hexachloraphane powder, the British government was left with little choice but to follow the American lead and ban its sale except in very dilute forms. Fortunately an alternative germicidal agent, chlorhexidine, is still available and is probably as effective for many purposes.

For obvious ethical reasons no final answer can be sought to the question of whether or not there is a genuine risk to human infants from the use of soaps containing 3 per cent hexachloraphane. Current medical advice is against its regular use in nurseries, and many hospitals have taken the simple way out and stopped its use altogether. Already there have been several outbreaks of bacterial skin disease in nurseries caring for newborn infants, and some of these have died. However, in the current climate of opinion there seems little chance of the ban being lifted.

A relatively new problem is inflammation of the genital area in women using aerosol deodorants. These are widely advertised among teenagers, and claims made suggest that only by the use of a vaginal deodorant can unpleasant body smells be removed. Cases have been reported in Britain and

America of irritative rashes in the genital area as a result of use of these sprays, and there have also been reports of skin reactions in male sexual partners of women using them. The current medical view is that deodorants should be confined to the armpits and that genital hygiene should rely on soap and water.

An allergic dermatitis may be caused by almost any substance that comes into contact with the skin. Metal objects often cause trouble, particularly the nickel plating of brassière clasps and suspender fastenings. Quite often rings, watches and spectacle frames also cause contact dermatitis, but the localized area of skin affected usually gives the necessary clue to the cause.

Less common – but also less likely to be incriminated – is dermatitis from cosmetics such as lipstick, the lanolin in face cream, the stretch nylon of tights or the dye inside a pair of shoes. Almost every type of clothing, cosmetic or jewellery has been responsible for a skin disorder at some time.

COSMETIC METAL POISONING

While allergic reactions to lipsticks and other cosmetics may cause unpleasant symptoms until the cause is identified, the condition is unlikely to be really serious. Such occurrences are rare and usually respond readily to treatment. Much more important for health are the cases of heavy metal poisoning that may be caused by some cosmetics used in Indian and African communities.

Surma is a grey powder applied to the eyelids with a thin wooden orange stick. The powder contains as much as 85 per cent lead sulphide and is highly poisonous. Punjabi families often smear this powder on the eyelids of quite young children – it is thought to benefit their health – and not surprisingly some of it often finds its way onto the fingers and so into the mouth and stomach. The powder is not on sale in Europe but apparently it is often brought into this country from India as a gift. Lead poisoning from this cause has been reported in children in the Punjabi communities of several cities in Britain.

The second group of potentially dangerous cosmetics are the skin-lightening creams, which have become popular in many East African countries. The danger from these creams became apparent only in the early 1970s when doctors at the University of Nairobi were puzzled by the fact that most of the adult patients with one type of kidney disease (nephrotic syndrome) were young, English-speaking African women. This curious selection suggested the possibility that a cosmetic might be responsible, especially as the nephrotic syndrome is known to be caused by poisoning with any of the 'heavy metals'. Tests showed that one of the most popular creams said to cause paling of dark skin contained up to 10 per cent of a mercury compound. Fortunately the kidney damage seems to be only temporary in most cases.

SUICIDAL SHAMPOOS

For some reason shampoos are occasionally swallowed by teenagers in a suicidal gesture after a quarrel with parents or a boyfriend. Ordinarily this does not cause serious symptoms, but it may be dangerous if the shampoo has been medicated for treatment of dandruff with the heavy metal selenium. This is a highly toxic substance, causing vomiting, loss of appetite and anaemia.

Selenium shampoos occasionally cause poisoning when used in excessive quantities on a scalp damaged by chronic skin disease such as eczema. The telltale symptom is a persistent odour of garlic on the breath.

CORSETS, GIRDLES AND SHOES

Mothers commonly tell their daughters that they will 'catch their death of cold' as a result of their choice of clothes; but this does not in practice seem to be a hazard of fashion.

One Western fashion is, however, thought to be responsible for much discomfort and misery: the corset or girdle. Though these are perhaps declining in popularity, millions of women still wear some sort of elasticated tube around their buttocks, squashing them into a desirable contour. There is good evidence that these tight garments are partly responsible for the prevalence of varicose veins in Western communities. This was strikingly demonstrated a year or two ago when Professor R. S. F. Schilling compared the health of 500 women cotton-workers in two mills in northern England with that of 500 working in five mills in Egypt. Whereas 72 per cent of the English women wore some type of corset or roll-on, only two (0·4 per cent) of the Egyptians did so; and over five times as many English women had varicose veins as the Egyptians. Furthermore, most of the English workers with vein abnormalities wore foundation garments.

Professor Schilling's work has since been confirmed by other doctors; and a 'pantie-girdle' syndrome has been described in which tingling and swelling of the legs are due to the wearing of too tight a girdle. The symptoms are likely to be made worse when a tight girdle is combined with a short skirt, since a girl then usually crosses her legs when she sits down, further constricting the flow of blood through her legs. In fairness to the fashion industry it should be added that Mr Denis Burkitt and other doctors have argued that the low prevalence of vein disorders in Egypt reflects the natural diet, high in bulk, eaten in that country and that the Western, refined diet is responsible for the high prevalence of vein disorders in Britain (see p. 52).

The other hazard of slavish attention to fashion comes from medically unsatisfactory shoes. Not many years ago the chief danger for both sexes came from the fashion for shoes with pointed toes. These necessarily squashed the toes together and in time a permanent deformity of the big toe – a bunion – was produced.

More recently this danger has receded; but the current

vogue for platform shoes is causing some medical concern. These shoes, sometimes with soles 6–8 in. thick, suffer from two design faults from a medical point of view. Firstly, the soles are flat; and it is a basic rule of good shoe design that they should either have a flexible sole or the sole, if rigid, should be rocker-shaped (as in the traditional wooden clog). If neither of these features is followed and the sole is flat and unyielding the wearer can walk only if the knees are kept bent. This throws an unacceptable strain on the ligaments around the knee, since the joint is fully stable only when locked in the straight position. Platform shoes have a second fault which adds to the first: they provide little support to prevent the ankle tipping over, and the height of the sole exaggerates the instability. Not surprisingly, orthopaedic surgeons have seen a minor epidemic of knee and ankle strains in fashion-conscious teenagers.

Whether or not the brassière is yet obsolete remains to be seen; certainly many teenagers now regard it as an old-fashioned relic of female subservience. The long-term effects of a bra-less society cannot yet be assessed, but it seems likely that they may include a greater demand for cosmetic surgery in the mid-twenties and early thirties, when loss of natural elasticity of the skin tends to lead to a pendulous bustline. This is because the breasts are not supported by muscle: their shape is the result of the interaction of the elasticity of the skin, the fibrous tissue beneath the skin and the form of the breast itself. Stretching of the skin and fibrous tissue as a result of lactation can lead to loss of shape, and so, perhaps, can handling during sexual play. While there is no scientific evidence that wearing a bra preserves the shape of the breasts, medical experts who believe that this is the case can claim support from the late Marilyn Monroe, who always wore a bra in bed.

SLIMMING

For the foreseeable future a slim figure seems likely to remain fashionable, so that slimming will continue to be a problem for women. So many books have been written on slimming that it is clear that no easy answer exists. It can be flatly stated that slimming drugs are rarely the answer and that some of them are dangerous (p. 224). As with stopping smoking, the crucial factor seems to be a genuine wish to succeed. Among teenage girls there is a danger that excessive preoccupation with losing weight may lead to the dangerous condition of anorexia nervosa. In this illness a girl (or very rarely a boy) virtually stops eating in an attempt to lose weight, and in severe cases the self-imposed starvation may lead to such severe loss of weight over a period of months that death results. The psychological causes of anorexia nervosa are not yet fully understood, but many experts believe that it starts with a subconscious rejection by a girl of her sexual development – she wishes to remain in the pre-pubertal state until she has come to terms with her own sexuality. Expert treatment early on is essential for any child who develops the disorder.

Chapter 10

ENVIRONMENT AND POLLUTION

OF the changes in our way of life in the twentieth century, perhaps the one most taken for granted – or not noticed at all – is the change in our atmosphere. The Edwardian Englishman spent his winter in Monte Carlo if his health was at all delicate, for in London and other big cities from November to March there was a succession of fogs against a background of rain and snow – and all of this when neither central heating nor double glazing was common. Control of atmospheric pollution has transformed the winter in industrial cities. London now has nearly twice as much winter sunshine as it did in the 1930s, and the change is even greater in cities such as Sheffield and Glasgow.

The abolition of industrial smog by the clean air legislation has been one major change in our climate, and its effect on health has been striking. Only comparatively recently have doctors begun to study scientifically the effects of environment on health, though some connection between the two has been accepted for thousands of years. Indeed, the father of medicine, the Greek physician Hippocrates, wrote a text *De Aere, Aquis et Locis* (*Airs, Waters and Places*), which discussed the medical merits of alternative environments.

Many of the traditional qualities of climates are based on no more than folklore. There is some general agreement as to which British seaside resorts could be described as 'bracing' and which as 'relaxing', but far less certainty about which is better for the health. Climates do influence diseases: so much so that some medical schools have separate departments of tropical medicine. In part this is due to the occurrence in tropical countries of infectious conditions such as malaria and sleeping sickness which are not found in

Europe unless brought there by travellers; but there are also specific conditions due to heat – prickly heat, sunstroke and heatstroke. Intestinal complaints are more prevalent in warm climates, and conversely cold, damp climates are traditionally associated with chest diseases as well as with chilblains and frostbite. Only since the application of formal scientific techniques in the science of epidemiology, however, has it been possible to separate the fact from the folklore and show which aspects of the environment in which people live truly affect their health.

BRONCHITIS

By far the most important health aspect of environment is the nature and extent of atmospheric pollution; industrial smoke, containing soot particles and sulphur dioxide, is the worst offender and the real danger to life. The most striking evidence of how lethal industrial pollution could be came in 1952, in the Great London Smog. This was an unlucky combination of meteorological circumstances which led to a dense fog persisting over the city for a week, made much worse by the smoke poured into it by millions of domestic fires and factory chimneys. Within seven days 4,000 people died.

Most of these were chronic bronchitics whose tattered lungs could not cope with the extra stress of filtering oxygen out of the dense soup-like atmosphere. Ten years later, between 3 and 7 December 1962 the atmospheric conditions were duplicated in another dense fog and 'inversion'. This time, however, there was far less smoke in the air, and bronchitics were warned by radio and TV to stay indoors; as a result far fewer died.

Not only has the clean air policy of the last twenty years got rid of the killer smogs: it is also well on the way to changing the pattern of illness in Britain. For most of this century, throughout the world doctors referred to chronic bronchitis as the 'English disease', since it was so much more common in Britain than other countries. Doctors argued that this propensity to bronchitis was a combination of the effects of the physique of the Englishman with his cold, damp climate. Only now is it becoming apparent that the responsible factor was the industrial pollution of the air of our cities.

Careful observation of bronchitics has shown that the rate of decline in their health is now much slower than it used to be. Laboratory measurement of lung function is based on the amount of air that can be taken into the lungs and the rate at which the breath can be expelled. The maximum volume of air that can be expelled from the lungs gradually declines with age, at a rate of about 25 ml. a year. Apparently bronchitics suffer a more rapid decline, and in Sheffield in the early 1960s this rate was shown to be about 85 ml. a year, based on 125 patients assessed regularly between 1960 and 1965. When the same tests were repeated on another group of 178 bronchitics between 1966 and 1972 the rate of decline had fallen to 25 ml. – the same as in normal persons. A few even improved their performance. According to Dr Peter Howard of the Sheffield University Department of Medicine, the only reasonable explanation for this change in the outlook for bronchitics is the change in the city's atmosphere. Between 1956 and 1972 the density of smoke particles in the air had dropped from over 300 μg./cu. m. to less than 40.

There is little doubt that bronchitis is more closely linked with atmospheric pollution than with climate. A study by the London School of Hygiene based on nearly 20,000 households in Britain showed that the prevalence of bronchitis correlated very closely with the density of smoke particles in the atmosphere. The second big factor in the causation of chronic bronchitis is, of course, cigarette-smoking (p. 243): but the survey showed that at every level of smoking the prevalence of bronchitis and its severity rose in proportion to the pollution of the atmosphere in the area concerned. Hence life-long non-smokers can apparently tolerate fairly high levels of atmospheric pollution without developing severe bronchitis, while people living in a clean atmosphere can smoke fairly heavily without increasing their risk of bronchitis by over about 20 per cent; but the combination of smoking and even low levels of pollution is dangerous, and heavy smoking combined with severe pollution may be lethal.

What of diseases other than bronchitis? Death rates from chest diseases in young children used to be higher in Britain than elsewhere in north-western Europe, and again there is good evidence that these diseases are more prevalent in areas with high atmospheric pollution. So much is this an effect of city pollution, indeed, that in a comparison of the health of country children in Australia, New Zealand and the United Kingdom the British children came out on top. Over 16,000 children were included in the study, in which their doctors were asked about the prevalence and severity of ill-health from hay fever, asthma and bronchitis. The only striking difference among the children was that hay fever and asthma seemed more of a problem in those parts of Australia with a hot, dry climate. The conclusion reached was that environmental factors – smoking, dust, industrial pollution and social conditions – are much more important in explaining the prevalence of disease than are climatic variations.

Some types of asthma, however, may be closely linked to geographical variations: those known to be due to a specific allergy. One common variant of allergic asthma is that due to a reaction to house-dust mites, and its relation to geography is an odd little medical detective story.

For over one hundred years Swiss doctors had observed that some (but by no means all) patients with asthma lost their symptoms on trips high into the mountains – and not unnaturally they attributed this improvement to the 'clear, pure mountain air'. This explanation did not, however, fit in very well with observations suggesting that there was a fairly clear line of demarcation at between 1,200 and 1,600 m. (3,500–5,000 ft). Then in 1967 Dutch research workers showed that many asthmatic patients were allergic to dust containing fragments of the house-dust mite, *Dermatophagoides pteronyssinus*, and that their symptoms disappeared if all traces of the mite were removed from their houses. The mite is usually found in damp conditions, most often in valleys and along the coasts of the North Sea. Tests on houses in Switzerland showed that there were few house mites in samples of dust taken in Davos (1,500 m.) – less than one fortieth of the concentration found in comparable houses in the Dutch town of Leiden, with its canals and damp climate.

INVISIBLE POLLUTION

This episode shows that the effects of climate on health are not necessarily direct. Indeed, now that the worst of the industrial smokes have been banned from the atmosphere of Britain and other countries there is mounting anxiety about the other, invisible pollutants of the air we breathe. 'Clean smoke' often contains high quantities of sulphur dioxide, and it seems that this gas is often dissolved by water vapour in the atmosphere to form sulphuric acid, with the result that rain falling downwind of large industrial complexes is sometimes quite heavily contaminated with acid. Fall-out of this kind has been blamed by farmers for poor crops and stunted growth of trees; the effects of acid atmospheres on human health have yet to be ascertained.

Of the invisible pollutants the best-studied are the oxidants responsible for the eye-smarting haze of Los Angeles, and the carbon monoxide and lead from vehicle exhausts present in the air of every city. Los Angeles smog first became a problem in about 1945, when it was noticed that during sunny weather the atmosphere became hazy and irritating to the eyes and nose. Research showed that this haze was due to a chemical action of sunlight on nitrogen oxides and hydrocarbons released from motor exhausts. The combination of physical and environmental features in Los

Angeles is probably unique – a high density of cars, low humidity, plentiful sunlight, warm climate and not much wind – and certainly no other city has had anything like the same amount of trouble despite the vast increase in the number of cars in all Western countries in the last twenty years. Nevertheless, the Los Angeles problem focused attention on motor exhausts as a cause of pollution and led indirectly to the current legislation insisting on tighter controls on vehicle emissions and on the lead content in petrol.

CARBON MONOXIDE

Carbon monoxide (CO) is at once the biggest and most dangerous pollutant in vehicle exhausts. In the USA motor vehicles release about 100 million tons of CO into the atmosphere each year, and it is the CO content of exhaust gases that makes them so lethal in a confined space. This century the amount of CO in the earth's atmosphere has risen steadily, to such an extent that environmentalists are worried about the 'greenhouse effect' by which the changed composition of the upper atmosphere retains more of the sun's heat, so raising the temperature of the atmosphere.

The health hazards of CO arise because it can combine with the red pigment in the blood, haemoglobin. During normal respiration the blood in the lungs is brought into close contact with the inspired air, and oxygen combines with the haemoglobin, forming oxyhaemoglobin. This is carried in the bloodstream to all parts of the body where the living cells need oxygen. In a rapid chemical action oxygen is exchanged for the waste-product carbon dioxide, and the blood returns to the lungs with its haemoglobin combined with the carbon dioxide. A further exchange is completed in the lungs, and so the cycle goes on. If the air breathed into the lungs contains any CO, however, then this combines with the haemoglobin more readily than does oxygen. The compound so formed – carboxyhaemoglobin – is very stable, and neither oxygen nor carbon dioxide can easily displace the CO from it. As a result even a very low concentration of CO in the air will lead to a gradual build-up in carboxyhaemoglobin in the blood. If the CO concentration is high eventually all the haemoglobin might be converted to the inert form – except that long before that happened you would be dead.

Breathing even as little as ten parts of CO in a million parts of air (10 p.p.m.) for twelve hours raises the carboxyhaemoglobin level to about 2 per cent, and a two-hour exposure to 50 p.p.m. will do the same. The effects of these small amounts of carboxyhaemoglobin are a matter of dispute among doctors. Unquestionably, people with 5 per cent carboxyhaemoglobin have impaired mental performance on arithmetical testing. Many authorities believe that levels between 2 and 5 per cent may be a major contributory factor in causing atheroma, the pathological condition responsible for coronary thrombosis and stroke (p. 298 and p. 301), the two main causes of death in Western society.

The situation is complicated by the fact that cigarette smoke contains rather more CO than does a car exhaust, so that a regular, heavy smoker who inhales may easily have a carboxyhaemoglobin level of 5 per cent or more. So more and more doctors now believe that the association between smoking and coronary thrombosis is a direct effect of the raised carboxyhaemoglobin levels in the blood of heavy smokers. If this is so then there might seem to be a health hazard for anyone whose work brought them into prolonged contact with traffic fumes. The carbon monoxide level of the air on an urban motorway is about 10 p.p.m. while it may rise to 50 p.p.m. in a traffic jam and levels of over 500 p.p.m. have been recorded in the Blackwall Tunnel, which carries traffic beneath the Thames.

Tests done on London taxi-drivers showed that those who smoked had higher carboxyhaemoglobin levels than non-smokers, but, once this effect was allowed for, the drivers on day shift (driving in dense traffic) had levels about 1 per cent higher than those on night shift. Some of the heavy smokers

among the day-drivers had levels as high as 10 per cent –
meaning that 10 per cent of their blood was useless for its
function of transporting oxygen. Similar results have been
shown for traffic policemen and others working in dense city
traffic.

Whether or not these differences in carboxyhaemoglobin
have long-term implications is a matter of opinion: non-
smoking taxi-drivers with levels of 2–3 per cent are in the
same range as moderate cigarette-smokers and so might be
expected to have the same risks of heart disease. Certainly the
view of the US National Research Committee on Effects of
Atmospheric Contaminants on Human Health and Welfare
is that there is no level of CO in ambient air without
effect.

LEAD IN THE ATMOSPHERE AND ELSEWHERE

After carbon monoxide, the constituent of vehicle exhaust
smoke that has given rise to most anxiety has been lead.
Petrol companies add lead to petrol (in the form of tetra-
ethyl lead) as an anti-knock agent. The presence of the lead
allows the motorist to use a petrol with a lower octane rating
than he would otherwise need, so that in practical terms
leaded petrol is cheaper. Between 7 and 30 per cent of this
lead is passed out with the vehicle exhaust, more at high
speeds than at low.

Usually lead from petrol is the most important single
factor accounting for lead in the atmosphere, and not surprisingly tests have shown that the atmospheric lead concentration is clearly related to the density of traffic. Because
emission of lead in the exhaust is related to throttle opening,
lead levels tend to be higher near urban motorways where
traffic is both dense and fast-moving.

Other sources of atmospheric lead may be important in
some localities. Several episodes have occurred of dangerous
amounts of lead being released into the air by smelters and

similar industrial plants (p. 155). In these circumstances a significant proportion of lead may be found in dust in the streets and houses in the vicinity.

Two other important sources of lead in the environment have caused anxiety in recent years: lead paint and lead water-pipes. Lead in paint comes from two sources: compounds used as pigments and the use of lead naphthenate as a drier. There is a statutory control on the use of lead paint for children's toys and furniture, but no other legislation governs the use of lead in paint. The practical problem arises because small children tend to chew objects in their environment, including banister-rails on staircases, window-sills and so on. Often they will chew all the paint off down to the bare wood, so that a house can be considered safe only if all layers of paint, old and new, are lead-free. Toys, cots and nursery furniture made in Britain must be painted with lead-free paints, but this is not always true of imported goods.

Another possible hazard in old buildings is the flaking of old paint, which may produce heaps of dust with very high lead levels. Lead was widely used for domestic plumbing in Britain until after the end of the Second World War, and many older houses still have lead-lined water-storage tanks as well as lead piping. Water dissolves metallic lead slowly; this effect is much more definite with soft water – its acidity increases the rate at which the metal is dissolved and the low calcium content of soft water impairs the formation of a scale of calcium carbonate on the inside of the pipe. Once this scale has formed – as it does rapidly if the water is hard – further action on the lead by the water virtually ceases. If lead and copper are both used for domestic piping, electrolytic action is almost inevitable at the joints, and this may lead to very rapid solution of the lead.

The World Health Organization has recommended a maximum lead content for drinking water of 0·1 p.p.m. with the rider that the lead content should not exceed 0·3 p.p.m. after sixteen hours' contact with the pipes. Much higher levels than these are sometimes found in old houses in soft-water areas in Britain, and within the last few years several cases of lead poisoning have been shown to be due to this cause.

Lead is a highly dangerous metal in the kitchen, yet it has been used for thousands of years because of its ease of working and resistance to corrosion. Lead containers are now little seen; but pewter is still widely used for drinking mugs and many earthenware jugs, basins and jars have a lead glaze. If these vessels are used for storage of an acid liquid such as cider then large quantities of lead may be dissolved and anyone drinking it is likely to be poisoned.

While exhaust fumes, industrial wastes, paint, glazed earthenware and water among them account for most of the lead in the environment, some lead occurs naturally in plants and in soils. There is some lead in many foods, and the average dietary intake varies between 100 and 500 microgrammes daily. Only a fraction of the lead in the diet is normally absorbed, though a further small quantity may be absorbed through the lungs if the atmospheric content is high.

Lead poisoning is one of the oldest of the environmental diseases of man. One theory of the decline and fall of the Roman Empire attributes it to widespread lead poisoning among the upper and middle classes as a result of the use of lead for plumbing and for cooking vessels. Acute lead poisoning is an obvious, painful illness due to ingestion of large quantities of lead. The most prominent symptom is pain – 'lead colic' – in the abdomen, usually combined with constipation. The victim, groaning in agony, is doubled up in pain, pallid, cold and sweating.

Much more common is chronic lead poisoning, caused by gradual absorption of lead as a result of industrial or automobile pollution. Again abdominal pain, colicky and griping, is one of the symptoms. There may be signs of damage to the nerves controlling muscles in the arms and legs – lead paralysis, typically causing weak wrist muscles. Anaemia is another common result of chronic lead poisoning, as is kidney damage.

However, frank signs of lead poisoning of this kind are not common. Most industrial concerns handling lead now carry out regular screening tests on their workforce to detect lead poisoning before symptoms develop.

There is much more concern about sub-clinical lead poisoning, especially in children. In the last few years many surveys have shown that young children in the worn-out, socially deprived areas of large cities commonly have raised blood-lead levels. Screening programmes in New York and Chicago have shown raised levels in 25 per cent of children, while in Britain similar results have been found in children living close to smelting plants and in the streets around motorway interchange areas – such as the notorious 'Spaghetti Junction' near Birmingham.

Doctors do not agree about the lead level which is dangerous for children, though they do accept that the figure of 80 mg./100 ml. (which is usually quoted as the safety limit for workers in industry) is far too high for small children. In children aged five or under there is some persuasive evidence that quite low levels may cause chronic brain damage and mental retardation. The cautious attitude taken by many paediatricians holds that no 'safe' limit can be set for blood-lead levels in children; in practice this means that children with over 40 mg./100 ml. will be given treatment to lower their level; with levels above 25 mg./100 ml. the source of the lead should anyway be sought and eliminated.

NOISE

Another form of pollution is noise – from traffic, aircraft, machinery or electronically amplified music. Recently it has become a common contention that noise may be harmful to health, and there is convincing evidence to bear this out.

Some industrial occupations are notorious for noise – boilermakers are known to suffer progressive deafness as a result of the fiendish clattering in their working environment – but not until 1972 was a workman awarded compensation from his employers for loss of hearing. In that case a propeller-shaper was awarded £1,250 on the ground that his employers had failed to provide adequate protection in the form of ear-muffs. However, deafness caused by noise at work is still not recognized as a prescribed industrial disease, so that to receive compensation a workman has to prove negligence on the part of his employers.

Lesser levels of noise also have an effect on hearing. Perhaps the most striking evidence is the negative study on Sudan tribespeople done by Dr P. H. Beales in the 1960s. He found a tribe of desert-dwellers to whom guns, traffic and even drums were unknown and showed that the acuity of their hearing between the ages of seventy and seventy-nine was equal to that of American men aged thirty to thirty-nine working in a noise-free environment. Almost certainly city-dwellers suffer some progressive impairment to their hearing as a result of daily exposure to the noise of traffic, while there is serious concern among ear-specialists at the effects on teenagers' ears of the noise levels common in discotheques. Industrial health recommendations generally assume that any workman regularly exposed to noise levels above 85 decibels should wear ear-protectors: yet discotheques and pop concerts commonly achieve noise levels of 100 decibels or more. (The decibel scale is logarithmic, so that an increase of 10 is a doubling of the loudness.) It seems that noise levels of 110 decibels for two hours may be expected to cause permanent hearing loss in about 16 per cent of people; and while at 100 decibels for two hours the risk is only 2 per cent, that is still considerable. 'It is a sad disability', said the *British Medical Journal* in 1970, 'for people to have their hearing impaired in youth to the level they might be resigned to expect at sixty.'

Environmental aircraft noise is rarely loud enough to cause permanent deafness, but it may have a cumulative, wearing effect on the nerves. Considerable interest was aroused in 1969 when London psychiatrists published figures showing that admissions to mental hospitals were more frequent in areas close to Heathrow Airport, where noise from aircraft was loudest. While the validity of this study has since been questioned there is no doubt that individuals whose sleep is disturbed by aircraft noise or other factors perform less well than might be expected at tests of intelligence and coordination. Sleep is disturbed more readily by sounds that have some significance for the sleeper – the cry of a baby disturbs a mother very easily – and it seems likely, therefore, that those residents of houses close to airfields who felt most aggrieved about aircraft noise would be those whose sleep was most disturbed by it.

The latest form of noise pollution to arouse public concern is infrasound – sounds of such low frequency that they cannot be appreciated as sounds at all by human ears. Infrasonic noise may be generated by machinery such as compressors and it may occur in vehicles travelling with the windows open, while apparently infrasound is common in large buildings, including factories, office blocks and hospitals. Infrasound may be clearly audible to persons with sensitive hearing, while in those who cannot hear it it may cause feelings of sickness and difficulty with breathing.

Some of the sensations experienced by audiences at pop concerts may, it seems, be due to infrasound. An article in the *New Scientist* has suggested that the discomfort, bad temper and other effects of thundery weather seen in susceptible persons may be due to infrasound. More information is being sought, but already an international conference in Paris has recommended 'acceptable' levels of infrasound for long-term human exposure: 120 decibels at 20 cycles/second rising to 140 decibels at one tenth of a cycle/second.

HARD AND SOFT WATER

In technically advanced countries each man, woman and child requires about 100 gallons (400 litres) of water each day. While most supplies are now bacteriologically pure, there are still big variations in their chemical content.

Hard water is so called because it leaves a hard, scaly deposit on the inside of the kettle or saucepan when boiled. The scale is formed from calcium and magnesium carbonates and sulphates, and these salts make it difficult to raise a lather with conventional soap. In contrast, soft water feels soft to the touch when used for washing and contains very much lower chemical content of salts.

Hard water was formerly associated with deficiency diseases, classically goitre, the swelling of the neck due to enlargement of the thyroid gland caused by lack of iodine in the diet. In most parts of the world the risk of goitre has been eliminated by adding small quantities of iodine to table salt. Some hard waters contain large amounts of fluoride, and indeed it is the normal health of people living in such areas that provides the advocates of fluoridation to prevent dental decay with the best evidence of the long-term safety of water with added fluoride (p. 42).

The big unsolved problem of water supplies is their effect on heart disease. Though it has been known for twenty years that people living in soft-water areas have a greater incidence of coronary thrombosis and related disorders than do those whose water is hard, it is far from clear whether the effect is due to a beneficial trace element in hard water or to a direct effect of soft water (p. 52).

Water-hardness affects the incidence of other disorders. Studies in the USA and Britain have shown that more babies are born with spina bifida (and other congenital defects of the brain and spinal cord) in soft-water areas. In spina bifida there is a failure of normal development of the bones of the spine and the underlying spinal cord. Affected children have some degree of permanent paralysis. More severe forms of the defect cause failure of brain development – anencephaly – which is always fatal. This problem was studied in detail in 1971 by the Welsh National School of Medicine, for within the relatively small area of South Wales there were no fewer than forty-eight local water authorities and the hardness varied between 39 and 161 parts per million. Within the South Wales area the rate of nervous system malformations per 1,000 births was shown to vary from about five to ten. The correlation between soft-water areas and high malformation rates was very striking.

These brain malformations are known to be more prevalent in families with a poor social and economic environment, and to some extent it could be argued that the soft-water areas of Wales are also the poorest. So the Welsh doctors separated their results into subgroups, of manual and non-manual workers, and still showed that the effect was there. A year later a bigger study by the London School of Hygiene suggested that any true association between these nervous-system malformations and soft water was small. The London work analysed the infant death rates from all causes in the sixty-one largest county boroughs in England and Wales. This showed fairly convincingly that infant mortality (ranging from 17 to 32 per 1,000 live births) was distinctly higher in soft-water areas than in those with hard water. The study was extended to include data going back to 1911, when the infant mortality ranged from 67 to 155, and the same relation was found to have applied. Most of the differences between different boroughs could be explained on the basis of known factors such as overcrowding, housing conditions and poverty; but it seemed that water-hardness made a contribution of 20–40 per cent of the differences in infant mortality.

One possible explanation for these findings might be the known tendency for soft water to dissolve lead out of water-pipes, and even in low concentrations lead might be dangerous to pregnant women. At present, however, there is no consensus of medical opinion on the significance of the link between soft water and birth defects – or indeed heart disease.

Sir George Godber was the chief medical officer of the Department of Health during the years when these discoveries were made and examined the reports as they appeared. He concluded in 1973 that it would be foolish at present to soften water-supplies further until the explanation is found for these associations. In practical terms anyone living in a hard-water area contemplating fitting a water-softener should make sure that the process does not affect the drinking-water supply drawn from the kitchen tap. On the other hand, the risks associated with soft water are small compared with those of smoking and overweight: certainly they do not justify anyone moving from a soft-water area on health grounds.

POLLUTANTS OF DRINKING WATER

In the United Kingdom water-softness and the associated risk of lead poisoning are the only important health aspects of the purity of municipal water-supplies. When water is taken from a spring or well, however, there are other hazards – in addition to the obvious one of bacterial contamination with typhoid and other organisms – such as pollution by nitrates from excess use of agricultural fertilizers. Nitrates may cause a form of anaemia, especially likely to affect babies. Other agricultural wastes may seep into sources of drinking water: interest has concentrated on organochlorine insecticides such as DDT, but since these compounds are only slightly soluble in water they have not been shown to constitute a real risk to health. In some areas of the world dangerous chemicals including arsenic, selenium and mercury are found in the soil and sometimes percolate into water-supplies.

WATER FOR RECREATIONAL USE

For the time being, at least, water authorities seem to be able to cope with increasing demands without sacrificing quality. By the time the water in the Thames reaches the sea, much of it has made several cycles – in which it is taken from the river, purified, passed into a water-supply, used by house-holders and factories, discharged to a sewerage plant and finally returned to the river. There are no medical objections to the use of 'second-hand' water, provided that the purification and testing processes are reliable. However, the accumulation of wastes in river, lake and sea water may cause considerable disturbance to its recreational use.

Careless disposal of human sewage is perhaps the most obvious cause of spoliation of water usage for recreation. While there are few aesthetic or hygienic objections to the discharge of treated sewage into rivers and coastal waters, some authorities still empty large quantities of raw sewage, quite untreated, into their local sea water. Reasonably enough, bathers and beachcombers object to the sight of lumps of sewage and toilet paper floating about in the surf; but there is no evidence that sewage on the beach is a source of disease. An investigation by the Public Health Laboratory Service in 1959 looked at infections in people using forty English beaches heavily contaminated with sewage. The conclusion reached was that transmission of diseases such as poliomyelitis, typhoid or paratyphoid is very rare even when beaches are heavily contaminated. The diluting action of the sea water probably immunizes the risk of infection, or it may be that very little sea water is swallowed by swimmers. The fact is that sewage in sea water has never been scientifically proved to be a serious health hazard, whatever the other objections that can be raised to it. 'Holiday typhoid' among visitors to the Mediterranean is much more likely to be due to eating contaminated seafood than to swimming in sewage-polluted water.

Again, industrial wastes are unlikely to be a direct hazard to swimmers: water which is aesthetically satisfactory for bathing is unlikely to be poisonous. Much more hazardous is the concentration of pollutants that may occur in fish and other marine organisms. The most notorious case was the outbreak of Minamata disease in Japan, where scores of people died and hundreds suffered irreversible brain damage from eating fish containing mercury, itself absorbed by the fish from industrial effluent discharged into the sea.

POLLUTANTS IN FOOD

Once the source of the outbreak of Minimata disease was identified in Japan there was a wave of interest in the possibility that other types of fish and indeed other foods might be dangerous. A temporary panic developed about the finding that most deep-sea tuna fish have mercury in their bodies approaching a concentration of 0·5 mg./kg.; but closer study showed that this concentration of mercury from sea water in the fish was a feature of the tuna's internal chemistry and nothing to do with industrial pollution. The mercury level of tuna fish is high: but it has almost certainly always been high and does no harm. People and animals who eat a lot of fish seem slowly to accumulate mercury but without any ill-effect.

Cadmium is another metal that seems to be concentrated by shellfish; those living in water polluted by industrial wastes may have 5,000 times the concentration of cadmium found in unpolluted waters, but no adverse effects have been recorded in those eating the oysters and clams. A specific disorder – itai-itai or ouch-ouch disease – was attributed to cadmium poisoning in Japan in the late 1960s. Undoubtedly there had been pollution of rice-paddies and water-supplies by waste from a cadmium-mining complex. The symptoms of the disease were due to multiple fractures in bones softened by a chemical change – osteomalacia – attributable at least in part to cadmium poisoning. However, since almost all the victims were women past the menopause who had had several children, it seemed likely that other factors were also involved.

WATER-BORNE PARASITIC DISEASES

The hazards of chemical pollution of water and fish are, in practice, trivial compared with the natural diseases that can be contracted from lakes and rivers. Two of the most important parasitic diseases still plaguing mankind are schistosomiasis (snail fever) and onchocerciasis (river blindness). Their names may be unfamiliar to most Europeans: but between them these two kill, blind or cripple millions of people every year in Africa and Asia, and over 250 million persons are thought to be chronic sufferers from these disorders. They are due to small parasitic worms or flukes which enter the body through the skin during bathing or wading in infected water. Unfortunately the new, man-made lakes of major hydroelectric schemes such as the Volta dam in Ghana have proved major sources of these infections, for which there are as yet not fully satisfactory medical or public health treatment programmes.

The role of stagnant water as a breeding-ground for mosquitoes is well-understood in parts of the world where malaria is a problem, and eradication campaigns have been successful, based on the use of DDT.

DDT AND PESTICIDES

Environmentalists have rightly drawn attention to the disastrous effects of DDT (and related organochlorine pesticides) on birds of prey. It seems that the effects on the birds' fertility are caused by the accumulation of high concentrations of DDT – birds of prey come at the end of the food chain. The most striking biological feature of DDT is its indestructibility: the stuff is chemically inert, and once put into the environment it remains there. Fortunately, perhaps, DDT is scarcely soluble in water, but it is readily soluble in fat and tends to accumulate in the fatty tissues of birds, fish and man. Some water organisms may have DDT levels 10,000 times that of the water in which they live.

DDT is readily detectable in human fat and for many years health authorities have measured its concentration in samples of fat taken at post-mortem from people dying of natural causes. The highest levels have been found in India and Israel, where DDT has been used very heavily. In the United Kingdom levels have been falling steadily in recent years, and there is no evidence that these sort of levels represent any hazard to health. Enormous levels have been recorded in workers exposed to DDT during their work – 1,131 p.p.m. in the liver of one man – without any symptoms or signs of poisoning. As with so many other chemicals or drugs under intensive investigation, there have been reports of liver tumours in mice exposed to DDT; but these findings may almost certainly be discounted in the light of the clean bill of health given by long-term studies of men working on malaria control in India. DDT has been widely used for over twenty-five years and – apart from its effect on bird predators – seems a remarkably safe compound.

NON-CLIMATIC EFFECTS

The effects on health of atmospheric pollution, climatic factors, and even the as yet unexplained relation of soft water to heart disease are susceptible to rational explanation. Some geographical features of disease remain an enigma and can only be described. Of these probably the best-studied is the effect of latitude on multiple sclerosis.

Multiple (disseminated) sclerosis is a fairly common disorder of the brain, spinal cord and nerves, usually coming on in late teenage or early adult life, and presently claiming 50,000 patients in Britain. The cause of the condition is unknown. Without apparent reason or any warning one or more parts of the body may become weak or paralysed, or lose all sensation; the vision may become blurred; or control over the bowels or bladder may be lost. These effects may last for a day, weeks or months when equally unpredictably some or all of the signs and symptoms may disappear.

Attacks may recur rapidly or be spaced apart by several years. Some patients have only one attack; others progress steadily downhill to death.

One of the few certainties about multiple sclerosis is its geographical variability. The closer a country is to the Equator, the lower the prevalence of multiple sclerosis; in Mexico, for example, the rate is only one thirtieth of that in Denmark, 60°N. of the Equator. There is also some evidence that the disease becomes less prevalent with increasing distance from the Greenwich meridian of longitude – Siberia has a much lower incidence than Scandinavia. Even more surprisingly, when people born in high-risk areas emigrate to a low-risk part of the world they take with them the risk prevalent in their native country – unless they emigrate in childhood, when the risk seems to be that of the country of adoption. In South Africa, for example, multiple sclerosis is much commoner in English migrants than in native-born South Africans, but English settlers who left Britain before the age of fifteen seem to have the same risk as South African whites.

Similar if less striking variations apply to many more common diseases. Some, like the differences in prevalence of cancer of the oesophagus, stomach, liver and intestines, are almost certainly due to variations in dietary customs. Others, like the unusually high prevalence of nasal cancer in southern China (but not northern areas of the country), are less easily explained. Cancer of the breast is relatively uncommon in Japan, but when Japanese move to California the prevalence of the tumour starts to rise after one generation and reaches levels similar to those in Americans within two generations. Again, as yet no explanation has been discovered.

FALL-OUT AND RADIATION

During the twentieth century mankind has been subjected to an increasingly wide range of sources of radiation: X-rays in hospitals and industry, nuclear power stations, nuclear weapons and the growing numbers of radioactive chemicals used in medical research and treatment.

Sometimes people forget that since its creation the earth has been bombarded with radiation from the sun and from 'cosmic rays' and that the earth's crust contains many naturally occurring radioactive minerals. Together these sources make up the background radiation against which the man-made hazards must be measured. Biologically, the effects of all the different types of ionizing radiation are hardly similar. Heavy doses cause radiation sickness, an acute illness with vomiting, skin irritation, falling hair and disorders of blood-clotting. The blood and the bone marrow are specially susceptible to the effects of radiation, and exposure to lower doses may cause no symptoms other than suppression of normal growth of the bone marrow and – more sinister – a change from normal marrow to one characteristic of leukaemia. Of the long-term ill-effects on the individual, indeed, the risk of leukaemia is much the most important, though other forms of cancer may be attributed to exposure to radiation, and there is also a recognized relation between radiation exposure and the development of cataracts in middle life.

These effects of radiation on the body are disturbing, but its actions on unborn children are even more so. Repeated studies have now proved the extreme sensitivity of the growing foetus to X-rays, and expectant mothers are now kept away from any source of radiation unless exposure is absolutely essential. Should X-ray exposure occur in early pregnancy there is an undoubted increase in the risk that the child will develop leukaemia or a related blood disorder in infancy – though it should be emphasized that this risk, though increased, is still very small.

The effects of low levels of radiation on the germ cells – ovaries and testes – are more debatable. Radiation is mutagenic, that is, it changes the genetic make-up of cells, which is then passed on to subsequent generations. These mutations may, of course, be beneficial as well as harmful, and in any case there is a steady 'natural' mutation rate (possibly linked to the levels of background radiation) that is essential for the process of evolution by natural selection. Unfortunately, however, many mutations are known to be recessive, which means that their effects may not become apparent for many generations; so that there is no way in which scientists can be certain of the extent, range and nature of any mutations that have occurred since the general increase in radiation levels this century. Reasonably enough, the attitude of authorities such as the World Health Organization has been to urge reduction of radiation levels so far as possible and, when there is unavoidable occupational exposure, to recommend screening of the sex glands, so minimizing the chances of later genetic effects.

However, since animals reproduce rapidly and have a shorter life-span than man, scientists can study the effects of radiation on many generations. On the basis of such studies the International Commission on Radiological Protection has laid down standards which seem reasonably safe. For example, the genetic dose limit for a whole population – taking background radiation into account – is recommended not to exceed 5 rem from all sources (a rem is the equivalent in any form of radiation of 1 rad of X-rays). If the mean age of child-bearing (male and female) is taken as thirty years this means that exposure from all sources, including background radiation, radioactive fall-out and medical X-rays, should not exceed an average of 0·15 rem a year.

Enough research has now been done to estimate the risks when these levels are exceeded. For example, in someone whose whole body exposure is as high as 0·5 rem a year the increased risk of leukaemia and other cancers is calculated as six to twelve cases of leukaemia per million individuals per year.

Against this background it is possible to see both sides of the argument about radioactive fall-out from tests of nuclear weapons. Atmospheric tests release into the stratosphere large quantities of radioactive dust particles. Some of these have short half-lives and so lose their radioactivity quickly, but others, such as strontium-90, are almost immortal. Fortunately, the short-lived components predominate so that by the end of 1967 over half the total of radioactivity released by the tests in the 1940s and 1950s had already been dissipated. Nevertheless, every additional test increases the amounts of 'immortal' contaminants. The implication of annual research studies is that the levels in current circulation have only a small effect on genetic mutation and the risk of diseases such as leukaemia; but at the same time it can be argued that no level is without some effect, so that no amount of fall-out can be described as safe. At present it is true to say that the level of radioactivity in the environment generally is declining – but critics of nuclear power stations point out that an accident in one of these large units could cause a major reversal of that trend.

Chapter 11

ALCOHOL AND DRUGS

ALCOHOL

ALCOHOL is almost certainly the oldest substance taken by man for its intoxicant effects. Every primitive people seems to have discovered the process of fermentation of sugar by yeast. The earliest alcoholic drinks were probably sugary fruit juices which had fermented spontaneously after being contaminated by airborne yeast spores. Fermentation of cereals to form beer is possible only if the grain is soaked to encourage partial germination. In its simplest form alcoholic fermentation comes to an end when the proportion of alcohol in the brew rises to somewhere between 10 and 20 per cent, since this concentration kills the living yeast organisms. Stronger drinks can be made only by distillation, and this vital step seems to have been taken after the fall of Rome; alcohol was first identified by Arabian chemists in Alexandria.

Indeed, it was the development of cheap distilled liquors that first led to major social problems from alcohol. Cheap gin became available at the same time as industrial overcrowding in Britain reached its worst levels, and the resulting conditions – 'drunk for a penny and dead drunk for twopence' – led to the first attempts by the government to curb drinking, spurred on by the Royal College of Physicians. The introduction of licensing regulations and a heavy tax on spirits certainly eliminated the worst excesses of nineteenth-century alcoholism.

In the modern world the amount of alcoholism in a society seems to depend on three factors: social customs, the affluence of the society and the price of drink. The league table for alcoholism is headed by France with an incidence of some 10 per cent of the adult population, compared with 3 per cent of Australians and about 1 per cent of Britons.

Society is concerned about excessive drinking for three reasons. Firstly, there is the social damage caused by alcoholism. The WHO definition describes alcoholics as

those excessive drinkers whose dependence on alcohol has attained such a degree that it shows a noticeable mental disturbance or an interference with their bodily or mental health, their personal relations and their smooth social and economic functioning or who show the prodromal [warning] signs of such development. They therefore need treatment.

Secondly, even if regular drinking does not lead to alcoholism it does expose the drinker to the risk of disorders such as cirrhosis, heart disease and stomach disease; and thirdly drinking is a major factor in causing road accidents, industrial accidents, violence in the home and broken marriages.

Nevertheless, total abstention from alcohol is rarely urged as a solution to its problems, despite the fact that this is the answer usually recommended for tobacco and other drugs such as cannabis. In most people's experience drinking is something they can take or leave alone – alcoholism is a problem that only happens to someone else. The National Council against Alcoholism estimates that of the British population of 50 million about 33 million drink, and about 20 million drink regularly. Perhaps 2–3 million drink heavily and therefore dangerously, and of these only half a million satisfy the WHO definition of alcoholism. What factors lead a social drinker to become an alcoholic?

Many aspects of addiction to alcohol are still unsolved problems, but it is now agreed by experts on the disease that there is no one single cause. The clearest demonstration of this is the age-distribution of alcoholics: the peak occurs in the range thirty-five to fifty-five, but alcoholics in their teens and twenties are by no means rare. The time that elapses from the age at which drink is first taken until the emergence of unequivocal symptoms of alcoholism may be anything between two and sixty years.

Some of the risk factors have been identified. Much has been written about the personality of the drinker who is likely to progress to alcoholism. The American view, first clearly developed by E. M. Jellinek, is that one form of alcoholism, alpha alcoholism, is primarily due to an underlying personality defect. Alpha alcoholics are introspective, socially immature individuals who often have sexual difficulties which prevent them achieving satisfactory adult relationships. It would be dangerously wrong, however, to suppose that all or even most alcoholics have clearly identifiable personality problems before they start drinking. The evidence strongly suggests that the majority of alcoholics were formerly apparently normal individuals whose behaviour was unexceptional. All that is needed for any drinker to become an alcoholic is a combination of availability and incentive to drink. Occupation, social class, age and marital status are all relevant to the risk of alcoholism. Heavy drinking is an almost inescapable hazard for publicans, journalists, public relations men and for many businessmen, and alcoholism is particularly prevalent in these occupations – beta alcoholism in Jellinek's system. In the age range fifteen to twenty-four married men have a higher incidence of alcoholism than do single; but in the peak age range for alcoholism, thirty-five to fifty-five, the problem is much more prevalent among single men. Apart from the obvious point that middle-aged single men are likely to have remained single on account of some personality problems, the fact that they are single makes it more likely that they have the time and money to spend in pubs and drinking clubs.

Drinking in children is being recognized as a growing problem in Britain. Alcoholics admitted to hospital in the 1950s generally gave seventeen or eighteen as the age at which they first took a drink; but a recent survey in London showed that 90 per cent of schoolchildren of both sexes have started to take an occasional drink by the age of fifteen, and there is a small but growing problem in big cities of drunkenness in schoolchildren as young as thirteen. Not surprisingly, admissions to hospital for alcoholism show a trend for an increasing proportion of men and women aged under thirty.

Alcoholism seems to be more of a problem at the extremes of social class than for skilled workers and the middle classes. Manual labourers often start heavy beer drinking in their teens as part of the accepted way of life among building workers and others whose job involves heavy physical exertion. At the upper end of the social scale heavy drinking is again an accepted feature of life in many families, money is available to pay for it, and its social effects are tolerated and concealed. Certainly among women alcoholism seems to be found almost exclusively at the extremes of social class.

The progression from social drinking to alcoholism may be slow or rapid; its most sinister feature is its gradual nature, so that at every stage the drinker believes that if he wishes to do so he could retrace his progress. Many of those in 'at risk' occupations find that they drink every day at lunchtime and in the evening, but believe that there is no problem since they never become really drunk. In fact their consumption of alcohol rises year by year and a very high proportion of such regular drinkers have become alcoholics by the age of fifty to sixty.

The biphasic association of alcoholism with prosperity and lack of it has become obvious in Britain in the last decade. As grinding poverty was eliminated in the late nineteenth and twentieth centuries working-class drinking became less of a problem; but the increase in material prosperity in Britain since the Second World War has seen a fresh rise in alcoholism. In the early 1950s the annual total of admissions for alcoholism to hospitals in England and Wales was less than 1,000; it is now approaching 10,000. Much of this alcoholism is among the middle and upper classes and is conducted 'genteelly'; convictions for public drunkenness have remained at about about 70,000 a year. The volume of alcoholic liquor drunk in the United Kingdom is rising steadily: while beer consumption has risen little faster than the population the amount of spirits consumed has doubled in the last ten years from 15 to 30 million proof gallons and that of wine nearly trebled from 20 to 60 million gallons.* National consumption is usually measured in litres of pure alcohol per person per year: on this basis Britain, with a consumption of about ten litres, is still well behind France, where the figure is nearer thirty.

Alcohol taken by mouth is absorbed rapidly, mostly from the upper small intestine. Drinks which contain more than 20 per cent alcohol are absorbed relatively slowly since they slow down the emptying of the stomach. The Scots know this very well, and to get a rapid effect from neat whisky follow it with a drink of beer.

Absorption of alcohol is delayed by food and by fatty drinks such as milk and olive oil. The blood concentration of alcohol after a drink depends on so many factors – whether food is in the stomach, the rate of stomach emptying, the size of the person taking the drink – that no reliable conversion tables can be devised to help a drinker estimate his 'legal level'. Furthermore, the regular drinker metabolizes alcohol more rapidly than the novice because his liver has adapted to it. Even so the maximum rate at which a normal-sized man can eliminate alcohol from the body is probably no more than 10–15 ml./hr. A man who has been drinking heavily until late at night may very easily still have a high blood-alcohol level the next morning.

Alcohol depresses and slows the function of the brain. As little as 50 mg./100 ml. in the blood is enough to impair

* The system used in Britain for measuring the strength of alcoholic drinks is archaic. Proof spirit is defined as that containing so much alcohol that it will not stop gunpowder from burning – a simple test that could be carried out aboard ship. In practice this means that proof spirit has over 57 per cent alcohol; most gins and whiskies are 70 per cent proof, which is roughly equivalent to 40 per cent alcohol. Wines contain 10–15 per cent alcohol, and beers up to 5 per cent.

driving ability, though in Britain the legal limit is set at 80 mg. As the level rises to 150 mg. or so most 'social' drinkers begin to feel a little unwell, and at 400 mg. most are unconscious. However, alcoholics may still be able to walk with levels approaching that figure. If enough alcohol is absorbed to lead to unconsciousness the drinker may die because breathing stops. Even small 'social' doses of alcohol reduce mental and physical efficiency. They also release inhibitions and suppress self-criticism, which is the explanation for the lubricating effect of alcohol at a party. Outside the brain, alcohol causes increased blood flow through the skin (leading to flushing), causes nausea, lowers the blood-sugar level, and in Shakespeare's words provokes sexual desire but takes away the performance.

Effects of alcohol on health

Even if heavy drinking does not progress to frank alcoholism it is likely to have other ill-effects on the health.

Stomach: Alcohol causes inflammation of the oesophagus and stomach; this is the explanation for the sensation of nausea the morning after a bout of heavy drinking. The inflammation of the stomach lining makes it more susceptible to other irritants: the combination of aspirin and alcohol is especially dangerous – it accounts for a high proportion of all cases of the potentially fatal condition of stomach haemorrhage.

Any regular drinker is likely to develop chronic inflammation of the stomach – chronic gastritis – and this explains the loss of interest in food. This may be further complicated by formation of a gastric or duodenal ulcer, but the incidence of peptic ulcers is not in fact significantly higher among alcoholics than the rest of the population.

Liver: The 'hobnail' liver of the chronic alcoholic used to be a star exhibit on the platform of temperance preachers, and undoubtedly this form of chronic liver disease is found most often in chronic alcoholics. Even among alcoholics admitted to hospital for treatment, however, the incidence of cirrhosis is only about 20 per cent, and among less heavy drinkers the risk is proportionately smaller. One important factor is the diet: a heavy drinker who eats a balanced diet may protect his liver from damage.

It seems likely that heavy alcohol consumption makes the liver more susceptible to damage from other sources such as infection and that this is the explanation for the link between alcohol and cirrhosis. Severe cirrhosis impairs blood flow through the liver, leading to a risk of internal haemorrhage, and to progressive impairment in the chemical functions of the liver. Once it is established, there is some evidence that the progress of cirrhosis can be halted by abstention from alcohol; but only too often the disorder leads to death from liver failure or from complications such as haemorrhage.

Heart: Only comparatively recently has it been recognized that alcohol can cause a specific form of heart disease, alcoholic cardiomyopathy, in which the heart muscle is weakened. This can lead to heart enlargement and so to failure of its pumping action. Cobalt, contained in some beers (though not in Britain), may also cause cardiomyopathy, but the condition is rare.

Vitamin deficiency: Alcohol is itself a carbohydrate food and most alcoholic drinks contain sugars and other nutrients, so that the heavy drinker finds that he needs less food. The chronic gastritis associated with regular drinking leads to an impaired appetite, and as a result of these two influences most heavy drinkers eat little food and what they do eat is rarely chosen for its vitamin content. Not surprisingly, therefore, vitamin deficiency is common. The most prominent deficiency is of vitamins of the B group (see p. 56).

Pregnancy: Perhaps the most recently discovered effect of chronic alcoholism is its action on unborn babies. Reports from North America suggest that women who go on drinking heavily during pregnancy may give birth to babies with a specific 'alcohol malformation': abnormal eyes, finger joints and skin creases in the hands associated with mental retardation (p. 287).

Alcohol and accidents

With experience, any regular drinker learns to disguise the effects of alcohol on brain function and muscular control. Nevertheless, research on the effect of alcohol on driving has shown that these effects are related to the dose, and that even a little alcohol in the blood – 50 mg./100 ml., equivalent to two small whiskies taken on an empty stomach – inevitably impairs performance in driving tests. It took many years of campaigning against vested interests before the public became convinced of the justice of convicting drivers on the basis of blood-alcohol estimations alone, but the beneficial effects of the introduction of the 'Breathalyser Act' are undeniable. Legislation ensuring conviction of any driver with a blood-alcohol level above 80 mg./100 ml. came into effect in Britain in 1967. The year before the Act the number of deaths in road accidents was nearly 8,000 and the total casualties nearly 450,000. The first year of operation of the drink laws cut death by 15 per cent and the total number of casualties by 10 per cent, despite a rise in the number of vehicles on the road. Although this legislation has now been in force for nearly ten years, a high proportion of all those killed in road accidents – particularly pedestrians – are found to have high blood-alcohol levels at post-mortem examination.

Alcohol is also an important risk factor in industrial and domestic accidents. Many people who fall down stairs do so when intoxicated, and this is true of the elderly as well as the young.

CANNABIS

The effects of alcohol are acknowledged in Western society but it is only in the Middle and Far East that its use is widely restricted or prohibited. In contrast, West and East have agreed about the need to control cannabis since 1922, when the League of Nations organized the second opium conference. The request that cannabis should be included in the list of narcotic drugs came from Egypt and Turkey; the Egyptian evidence stated that

taken in small doses hashish perhaps does not offer much danger, but there is always the risk that once a person begins to take it he will continue. He acquires the habit and becomes addicted to the drug, and, once this has happened, it is very difficult to escape ... addicts in Egypt always return to their vice. They are known as 'hashashees', which is a term of reproach and in our country they are regarded as useless derelicts.

More recently this traditional view of cannabis as a dangerous addictive drug has been challenged, and there has been considerable pressure in North America and Western Europe to modify the legal restrictions on its use. Few subjects have aroused such strongly held opinions than the dispute about the risks, if any, attached to use of the drug.

Cannabis is a flowering plant, Indian hemp (*Cannabis sativa*). The dried leaves of the plant are termed 'marihuana' or 'dagga', and a resin obtained from the flowers is called hashish. In Western society a constantly changing range of slang terms are used to describe cannabis derivatives, but the most consistent is 'pot'. Whatever form of the drug is used (the commonest custom in Europe is for it to be smoked), the active ingredients seem to be a group of chemicals called tetrahydrocannabinols.

The effect of smoking cannabis comes on within thirty minutes and lasts for several hours. If cannabis is eaten there is an interval of up to three hours before its full effect. The immediate physical actions of cannabis are relatively minor: there is some reddening of the eyes, a fall in blood pressure and a rise in the heart rate. Cannabis depresses liver enzymes, and as a result it prolongs the sleeping time after barbiturate sleeping pills. The striking effects of cannabis are its psychological ones. Reactions to it are varied, and seem to be more obvious if the drug is taken in company, but the two most consistent are euphoria – a feeling of well-being – and a change in response to external stimuli, so that colours, sounds and social intercourse appear more intense and meaningful. Time changes: a subject who had taken cannabis typically responds too early when asked to estimate the length of a minute. Performance at tests of mental arithmetic and at simulated driving tests become impaired, and this effect becomes more noticeable as the dose increases. Recent memory and selective attention are both impaired – someone high on cannabis may give the impression that he has not heard what has been said to him.

Professor W. D. M. Paton, of Oxford University, who has done a great deal of research on cannabis, believes that the psychological effects of cannabis can be explained by the theory that it removes a restraining gate on the inflow of sensory information. Normally the brain ignores sensory stimuli that are either familiar or apparently irrelevant. Removal of this selection process leads to the flood of sensation that occurs with cannabis. The time sense depends on the frequency of sensory impressions, and an increase in the flow of these impressions would necessarily give a false impression of time. The effect of cannabis on memory would also be explained. Something which might be memorized needs either conscious or unconscious repetition if it is to be transferred from the temporary short-term memory state to the permanent memory banks. This conversion of short-term to long-term memory is interrupted by an increased flow of sensations – just as a telephone number may be forgotten if someone speaks just after it has been given. The increased flow of sensory impressions under cannabis probably interferes with the consolidation of recent information in a similar way.

All the psychological effects of cannabis seem to be controllable to some extent by the drug-taker. The intensity of the response can be reduced by a conscious wish to return to normal, and conversely even a small dose can have an appreciable effect if taken in a group all of whom wish to experience maximum sensations.

Even the opponents of cannabis would concede that there is a negligible physical or mental hazard from a single exposure to the drug. The Home Office Advisory Committee on Drug Dependence, reporting in 1968, agreed with the earlier reports of the New York Mayor's Committee and the Indian Hemp Drugs Commission that even regular consumption of cannabis in moderate dosage seems to have no harmful effects. So why are there still restrictive laws?

In part the answer lies in the vast amount of anecdotal evidence from countries with long experience of cannabis derivatives. The North African and Arab countries where the drug is grown – and has been for centuries – retain their view that it can destroy those who become dependent on it. No really long-term studies of the effects of cannabis on man have been done in Western countries to contradict this view, and the research on animals has merely shown that the drug is remarkably non-toxic in high dosage. Furthermore, as the drug has become more widely used in the West evidence has begun to accumulate of its ill-effects. The history of addictive drugs in the twentieth century is repetitive: cocaine, pethidine and amphetamine are all examples of drugs that were said to be free of serious risk of addiction when they were first introduced – and they are certainly less addictive than heroin or opium. Cannabis may well prove to be even less addictive than amphetamine or pethidine, but there is evidence now that psychological dependence to it does occur, and this is the classification given to it by the World Health Organization. Some regular cannabis smokers become dependent on it in exactly the same way as a proportion of regular drinkers become alcoholics. How high this proportion is is still not known, nor is it known how long the progression to dependency takes to develop.

Cannabis differs from narcotic drugs such as heroin in that definite tolerance does not develop. Instead, like the familiar nicotine, a regular cannabis smoker fairly soon establishes a dose that satisfies him and this dose does not then increase further with time. The dependence that develops is a psychological dependence – the smoker has a powerful wish to maintain regular consumption – again in the same way as a tobacco-smoking nicotine addict (p. 251).

The big argument about cannabis is the effect of long-continued heavy consumption. Opponents of use of the drug claim that it induces an 'amotivational syndrome', characterized by apathy, loss of interest in any purposeful occupation, social passivity and deterioration. This is the condition traditionally attributed to cannabis in Eastern countries, and undoubtedly such a picture is seen in regular cannabis smokers in the West; but the cause–effect relationship has not been proved. One of the difficulties in establishing the role of cannabis in this syndrome is that almost all sufferers have taken substantial quantities of other drugs as well – particularly heroin, amphetamines and barbiturates. Current sociological attitudes in Western society are such that anyone who rejects traditional values and 'drops out' is likely to smoke cannabis. Is his lack of motivation due to cannabis or is cannabis smoking a sign of rejection of conventional motivations?

More serious is the suggestion that cannabis may harm the brain. The tetrahydrocannabinols – the active principles of cannabis – are fat-soluble, and in animal experiments these compounds accumulate in fatty organs including the brain and the sheaths of the nerves. To some extent tetrahydrocannabinols have a cumulative effect; excretion of an absorbed dose is very slow. In 1971 the late Dr A. M. G. Campbell and his colleagues in Bristol shocked the pot-smoking world by reporting in the *Lancet* that this accumulation of cannabis metabolites in brain tissue could in time permanently reduce the size of the brain. The physical changes they described in the brains of ten young men who had all taken cannabis regularly for some years were such that they could explain the amotivational syndrome.

The report aroused a storm of controversy on both sides of the Atlantic. No direct confirmation of Campbell's findings has yet been published, and at present the case for chronic brain damage from cannabis remains unproved.

In 1975 the psychiatrist at Bir Hospital in Katmandu reported in the *British Journal of Psychiatry* that regular cannabis-users in Nepal had a poor work record, poor social and family relationships, and lack of interest in sex and a general loss of initiative and efficiency. Their conversation was monotonous and vague; they spent most of their time sleeping or sitting and day-dreaming. 'It is surprising', wrote Dr Sharma, 'to see how a person can spend time idly, not only for days but for years together.' He found no evidence of permanent physical effects, however: on the few occasions when he persuaded a heavy addict to give up cannabis, both physical and mental health had returned to normal within four months.

For the time being, the health authorities in most Western countries have decided that on balance the risks of legalizing cannabis outweigh any possible advantages. It is not valid to argue that alcohol or tobacco are more dangerous: the reason they are not banned on health grounds is simply that the only recent attempt to ban either in a Western country – prohibition in the USA – was a social disaster.

DRUG-TAKING AND ADDICTION

Drug-taking by schoolchildren and teenagers has become a major social problem in Western countries only in the last fifteen to twenty years. Addiction to heroin, morphine or cocaine has been recognized since de Quincey's *Confessions of an English Opium Eater*, but widespread use of medical drugs for stimulant effects by adolescents at week-end parties was a new development in the 1950s and early 1960s. The first group of drugs to be abused in this way were the amphetamines. These drugs – Benzedrine and Dexedrine are examples – stimulate mental activity, reduce fatigue and depression, prevent sleep and reduce the appetite for food. For a time in the late 1950s amphetamines were thought to cause little harm when taken as 'pep-pills' and were also widely prescribed by doctors for middle-aged housewives who had trouble losing weight. By the time the risk of addiction had been recognized there were tens of thousands of patients dependent on amphetamines. In the mid-1960s over 3 million NHS prescriptions were issued each year for amphetamines and there were estimated to be 150,000 addicts. So serious was this situation that the medical profession itself imposed a voluntary ban on prescribing these drugs; most experts consider them to have little role in treatment anyway.

In the 1960s a vast number of other drugs came to be used illicitly. Some, like the barbiturates, had been in medical use for many years without causing serious problems of addiction – though there were, and no doubt still are, millions of respectable citizens who would not give up their sleeping-pills; other drugs, like Preludin and Durophet, were introduced as 'safer' alternatives to amphetamine. Furthermore, with the growing popularity of mysticism as an alternative to orthodox religion, psychedelic drugs, especially mescaline and lysergic acid, were widely used for their effects on the mind, while there was an enormous growth in interest in cannabis. By the mid-1960s drugs had become an accepted feature of teenage life in Britain, and to the 'soft' drugs – amphetamines, barbiturates and cannabis – were added the hard drugs heroin and cocaine. Furthermore, even those addicts who knew enough to stay off heroin began to turn to intravenous use of soft drugs. Government action took the form of legislation tightening controls on the possession, prescription and distribution of the various groups of drugs. It now seems that the drug problem in Britain may not be getting any worse and could be easing.

The central principle of management of drug-addiction in Britain has been that addiction itself is not an offence. Any drug-addict may be supplied legally by a doctor provided that he at least tacitly accepts a need for treatment. In the case of hard drugs prescriptions can be given only at an authorized treatment centre. Cannabis is never prescribed – but addiction to cannabis is said not to occur, only psychological dependence. The success of this policy is shown by the official Home Office statistics. During the middle 1960s the numbers of known addicts to heroin and related drugs rose steadily year by year, reaching a peak of 2,881 in 1969. Since then there has been a slight decline, and indeed the number of teenage addicts has fallen sharply. These figures seem to imply that fewer young people are being introduced to heroin. Black-market heroin – much of it illicit 'Chinese' heroin – is of very doubtful purity and quality and is recognized as dangerous by addicts themselves. Though the Home Office figures refer only to registered addicts, there is no reason to believe that there are many unregistered; very few of the steady procession of heroin addicts admitted to hospital with jaundice, blood-poisoning, and other complications of the condition turn out to be unregistered.

Medical concern about drug-addiction is based partly on its disruptive effect on psychological development and partly on its physical hazards. The philosophy of the drug-addict may have developed independently and may be a cause rather than a result of his addiction; that argument has yet to be settled. Certainly there is abundant evidence that teenage drug-abusers tend to come from broken homes and to have other features of a 'disadvantaged environment', and this may partly explain the link between drugs and crime. More likely is the practical explanation that drug-addicts need to steal to eat: they can rarely hold a regular job and if they have no fixed address are not eligible for social security benefits.

There is little dispute about the physical hazards of drug-addiction, which are of course most definite with heroin. The death rate for young drug-addicts is horrifyingly high: a heroin-addict who relies on illegal supplies probably has a life expectancy of less than three years. Death may occur from overdosage – especially if the addict mixes drugs with alcohol. Overdosage is more likely if the addict relies on illegal supplies, since the strength of their heroin varies from one consignment to the next. Death may be due to hepatitis – inflammation of the liver caused by a virus which is transmitted when addicts share a needle or syringe that has not been adequately sterilized. Blood-poisoning from dirty needles or contaminated drugs is another risk; while the addict's poor diet lowers his resistance to a whole range of diseases from pneumonia to skin infections.

Chronic kidney disease leading to renal failure is also unusually common among heroin-addicts, but the cause of these kidney lesions is still unknown. They may simply result from recurrent bacterial infections associated with the use of dirty needles; or it may be that heroin (like mercury or phenacetin) is a kidney poison. Long-term follow-up of narcotic addicts is difficult, since they tend not to be regular in their habits. One such survey done in the King's Road area of London showed that of 108 addicts followed for seven years, twenty-five were off drugs, thirty-five were still being prescribed drugs in a recognized clinic, twenty-nine might not have been still taking drugs, and nineteen were dead. Reliable statistics are available about deaths, since they are usually investigated at an inquest.

In a series of deaths in narcotic addicts analysed by a London addiction expert, Ramon Gardner, ninety-seven were due to accidental overdosage; twenty were attributed to suicide (several killing themselves in prison); twenty-four died from infections including hepatitis and blood-poisoning; twelve died from natural causes – heart disease, asthma or diabetes – to which the narcotic addiction may have contributed; nine died in accidents such as drowning; six died from complications of treatment; and two were murdered.

Drug-addiction has now been repeatedly shown to behave as if it were an infectious disease. A single teenage addict may pass on the habit to fifty others within a few weeks, especially in a community with the social conditions known to promote drug problems. It is the combination of high mortality and this infectious nature of addiction that justifies public health measures to control it. Mental illness associated with drug-taking is mainly a problem with psychedelic agents – though acute psychosis may be caused by overdosage of amphetamines. Undoubtedly the most dangerous drug from this point of view is LSD (lysergic acid). Even its advocates admit that the effects of 'acid' are unpredictable; anyone taking a single dose may have a frightening, unpleasant hallucinating experience lasting several hours (a 'bad trip'). Less often abnormal mental reactions may recur hours, days or even weeks after exposure to the drug, and in the absence of restraint the victim may for example jump from a high window in the mistaken belief that he can fly. An acute panic reaction is sometimes seen as a reaction to cannabis, almost always in someone with little experience of the drug. Very occasionally acute psychosis has been attributed to cannabis: for example, delusions of persecution leading to violence have been reported among American servicemen in Vietnam, but possibly the drug used was contaminated. The amotivational syndrome associated with prolonged heavy use of cannabis is socially the most threatening of the effects of illegal drugs, but its existence is still denied by many authorities on marijuana.

Some of the less-used intoxicants have their own dangers; for example, teenagers periodically rediscover the fact that aeroplane glue has an intoxicating effect when sniffed, and inhalation of dry-cleaning fluids has also been fashionable intermittently. In each case the volatile agent responsible for the effect is a heavy hydrocarbon similar to chloroform or ether. Glue-sniffing is highly dangerous: many deaths have been recorded, usually from sudden heart-failure, since these hydrocarbons (even in relatively low dosage) irritate the heart muscle and can change the regular heartbeat into rapid irregular beats which can cause death very quickly. Glue-sniffing can also cause death or serious illness from damage to the liver or kidneys.

WHO TAKES THE DRUGS?

Statistics on soft-drug-taking in Britain are difficult to obtain, but some trends are obvious. Cannabis is certainly very widely used, especially among students. Convictions recorded by the Home Office for possession of cannabis were fewer than 5,000 in 1969 but had doubled by 1972 and still seem to be rapidly increasing. Almost certainly several million people in Britain have now committed technical offences associated with cannabis. Drug offences concerned with barbiturates and other agents apart from cannabis have also increased in the last few years, but at a much lower rate. The total number of convictions for all kinds of drug offences (embracing heroin, amphetamines, cannabis, barbiturates and all other controlled drugs) was over 16,000 in 1971, 20,000 in 1972 and 23,000 in 1973.

DRUGS AND ATHLETICS

At much the same time that teenagers began taking amphetamine pep-pills, athletes discovered their potential for relieving fatigue. No serious scientific evaluation has ever been made of the value of stimulants in athletics, but in addition to their known action in postponing the need for rest or sleep many sportsmen believe they improve their energy output and reduce awareness of pain. Not surprisingly their use became widespread, especially in endurance events such as long-distance cycling. In addition to the manifest unfairness of the use of drugs in sport they have real dangers – and deaths have occurred from a combination of exhaustion, heat and drugs, including one notorious case of a professional cyclist in the Tour de France. All national and international sports agencies now ban the use of drugs, and with improved methods of testing blood and urine specimens the use of stimulants has declined in recent years.

No reliable test has yet been devised that can detect the use of anabolic steroids. These drugs are chemically related to the sex hormones and their use increases muscle bulk. A course of anabolic steroids lasting a few months can help a shot-putter or weight-lifter gain 50–100 lb., and this may make a critical difference to his performance. Indeed in the last decade there has been a noticeable increase in the size of international-class athletes in the field events (shot, discus and javelin) and in weight-lifting, and probably almost all have taken anabolic drugs; but detection is unlikely since the drug can be stopped a few days before any important competition when chemical tests may be called for.

Anabolic steroids are undoubtedly dangerous. As with any other hormone-like drug, prolonged use interferes with the normal hormone balance of the body and may lead to secondary impotence. More important is the effect of anabolic steroids on the liver. These drugs have been used since the mid-1960s in treating some forms of anaemia, and at least five cases of liver cancer have been reported in patients on long-term treatment with oxymetholone, methyltestosterone or methandienone. While no case of liver cancer has yet been reported in an athlete treated with anabolic drugs, some degree of liver damage is common, and if a fine needle specimen of liver is examined a predictable pattern of abnormality can be seen under an electron microscope. A similar pattern is sometimes seen in women treated with oral contraceptives.

Pain-relieving drugs may also be abused in sport. A top-class athlete may take part in no more than a handful of really important events in a year, and there is a grave temptation for him or her to seek medical help to be fit for the big day. Combinations of pain-relieving drugs and anti-inflammatory agents may be given by injection into a damaged or strained tendon or muscle, and this will give a few pain-free hours. The risk is that abolition of the natural warning mechanism of pain may lead to permanent damage to the injured limb. Oddly enough, the use of drugs of this kind is illegal for race-horses but not, it appears, for athletes.

Any athlete who takes drugs prescribed for a chronic disability such as eczema should take reliable advice on their permissibility in his sport. In the 1972 Olympics an American swimmer, Ricky DeMont, was disqualified because he had taken a standard asthma remedy, ephedrine sulphate, which is related to the amphetamines. Permissible alternatives are nearly always given to an athlete who needs regular medical treatment.

Chapter 12

TOBACCO SMOKING

TRADITIONALLY 'Sir Walter Raleigh was the first that brought tobacco into England and into Fashion,' as John Aubrey tells us in his *Brief Lives*, adding that he took a pipeful to calm his nerves before going onto the scaffold; yet the Aztecs had smoked tobacco for several hundred years before Spanish explorers brought back the habit to Europe in the sixteenth century. In Britain tobacco became so popular that a tax was imposed on it in 1590. After a decline in the next century, it returned into favour in the 1700s, when doctors started to recommend it as a disinfectant and for treating various illnesses.

Until the Crimean War most people in this country smoked pipes or took snuff, but soldiers who had fought in the Crimea introduced the continental habit of cigarette smoking. By the time of the First World War cigarettes were accounting for half of all the tobacco smoked. Women also began to smoke during the First World War and the 1920s, so that the total amount of tobacco smoked rose steadily to a peak in 1945, when an average of twenty cigarettes were being smoked every day for every adult in the country.

Immediately after the Second World War tobacco consumption fell sharply. It had to be paid for in hard currency and was relatively difficult to get, while the new civilians who had had an allowance of cheap cigarettes in the forces suddenly found them expensive and needed their money to set up home. So tobacco consumption did not rise again until the 1950s, and since then it has risen and fallen, hovering around the level reached as far back as 1914. The primary reason for this low level, however, has probably been the publication of a series of reports on the link between smoking and serious diseases.

Although some doctors had suggested that cigarette smoking was connected with premature death or with lung cancer as far back as 1937 and 1941, respectively, other doctors had pooh-poohed these theories. It was not until 1950 that two British research workers, Sir Austin Bradford Hill and Sir Richard Doll, established both links by careful statistical analysis. Their work was confirmed by research in many countries, and other studies showed links between smoking and bronchitis, coronary heart disease and tumours of the urinary system, as well as an effect on the unborn baby (tending to make it significantly lighter in women who smoke during pregnancy).

The results of all this research were summarized by the Royal College of Physicians of London in two comprehensive reports. (This chapter owes much to the second report, *Smoking and Health Now*, published in 1971.) In the USA a similar report was published by the Surgeon General in 1964. The Chief Medical Officer of the Department of Health in London has also reiterated the serious dangers of tobacco smoking in his annual reports, while in 1971 the organization ASH (Action on Smoking and Health) was formed to tell the public about the dangers of smoking and to try and reduce them.

These reports and the ASH project have been widely publicized in the press, radio and television, and virtually every adult in Britain must now know that smoking has been connected with certain serious diseases. Such knowledge has had several effects. Some people have stopped smoking altogether – particularly doctors – so that by 1972 there were as many non-smokers as smokers. For the first time the distribution of smokers showed a definite social bias, relatively more manual and unskilled workers smoking than people in the professions. Tobacco consumption in this country is now tending to fall – a trend seen elsewhere only in the USA – and with our annual consumption of 5·9 lb. of tobacco per adult (equivalent to about 3,250 cigarettes) we are twelfth in the world smoking league, below all the developed countries except France and Greece. Total tobacco consumption has also fallen because of the increased popularity of cigars (which are smoked in smaller quantities) and the extensive switch to smoking filter-tipped cigarettes (1 per cent of all cigarettes smoked in 1950, compared with almost 75 per cent in 1971), though there is no evidence that the latter change has come about because of fears about health.

Despite all these trends, more than half the adults in Britain still smoke, and every year there are at least 50,000 deaths attributable to smoking in men and women aged 64 or less. The rest of this chapter summarizes what we know about the chemical make-up of tobacco smoke, why people smoke, the various risks they run and methods of stopping.

CONSTITUENTS OF TOBACCO SMOKE

Tobacco smoke contains at least 1,000 substances, depending on the type of tobacco – not only the different types in cigarette, cigar and pipe tobacco, but also the various forms used in the different brands of cigarettes themselves. Much recent research into this aspect has enabled scientists to construct 'league tables' classifying cigarettes by how much of some of the main constituents they contain. Smoke consists largely of tiny oily droplets suspended in air and contains four main types of substances: nicotine, tar, irritants and carbon monoxide. There are also traces of several other substances, such as arsenic and cadmium, which are thought not to have much effect on the body.

The action of nicotine is largely due to an initial stimulation of the central nervous system, followed by depression. In people unused to smoking stimulation of part of the brain may cause vomiting, but in habitual smokers (apart from a mild calming effect) nicotine mainly affects the heart and circulation. These effects are caused by the release of more adrenaline and noradrenaline, hormones from the adrenal glands: these make the blood pressure rise slightly, the blood-vessels in the skin narrow and those in the muscles widen, and the heart beat slightly faster and work harder. Nicotine also has two actions which may make smokers more liable to develop atheroma (p. 44): it raises the level of fatty acids in the bloodstream, and increases the stickiness of the platelets in the blood – cells which play an important part in blood-clotting.

The nicotine content of a cigarette varies from under 0·3 mg. to 3.2 mg. Those who inhale cigarette smoke may absorb up to 90 per cent of the nicotine, compared with 10 per cent in non-inhalers. Pipe and cigar smoke are more irritant, and so are less commonly inhaled, smokers absorbing some nicotine from the inside of the mouth. This is easier because pipe and cigar smoke are alkaline, enabling nicotine to be absorbed more readily than if it is in an acid smoke, as produced by cigarettes. Though pipe and cigar smoke contain more nicotine than cigarette smoke, pipe and cigar smokers absorb only a third as much into the bloodstream as do cigarette smokers who inhale.

The second main constituent of tobacco smoke, 'tar', is the yellow-brownish substance that condenses from tobacco smoke. Painted repeatedly on the skin of laboratory animals, this tar produces tumours, while analysis shows that it contains at least twelve substances known to cause cancer. Both cigar and pipe smoke contain more tar than cigarette smoke, and are more effective in producing skin tumours in mice; cigarette filters reduce the cancer-producing tendency of the tar.

The third main constituent is the irritants. Though cigar and pipe smoke are more irritant than cigarette smoke, within three minutes of inhaling cigarette smoke the air passages become narrower, probably because of the carbon particles in it: a smoker takes at least ten times as many particles into his lungs as the average non-smoker living in a city such as London. This narrowing of the air passage, which is significantly diminished if filter cigarettes are smoked, is too slight to be noticed by the average person, though the athlete would notice it as impaired 'wind'. Irritants also provoke coughing and slow down the action of the cilia – fine, hair-like projections from the cells lining the air passages, which normally help to remove substances inhaled into the lungs. Besides carbon particles, other irritants include phenols, aldehydes and cyanide – some of which increase the cancer-producing activity of tar.

Tobacco smoke contains about 5 per cent of carbon monoxide (CO), the gas which used to be the main constituent of town gas. If inhaled, CO readily diffuses through the lungs and combines strongly with some of the haemoglobin in the red blood cells. This interferes with the normal function of haemoglobin, which is to transport oxygen from the lungs to the rest of the body. The concentration of this carboxyhaemoglobin (COHb) is lowest in the morning before smoking, and tends to rise throughout the day; heavy smokers (fifty cigarettes a day) may have levels as high as 10–15 per cent. Once the person stops smoking, the COHb concentration falls to about half within two and a half hours, particularly if he takes some exercise. After smoking the same number of cigarettes, women show a greater rise in COHb than men, probably because their blood contains less haemoglobin with which the gas can combine.

Inhaling tobacco smoke has a considerable effect on the amount of CO absorbed into the bloodstream. In life-long pipe and cigar smokers, COHb levels are little different from those in urban non-smokers. But in cigarette smokers who switch to pipes or cigars the level remains much the same, presumably because they go on inhaling. In a pregnant woman who smokes, the COHb levels in the unborn baby may be double that in the mother, possibly because the different type of haemoglobin which is found in the embryo's blood takes up CO more avidly than adult-type haemoglobin.

Normally the blood of smokers contains too little COHb to cause any symptoms of CO poisoning (flushing, severe headaches, dizziness and unconsciousness), since these do not occur until concentrations of 30–50 per cent are reached.

Even so, when the amount of oxygen in the air is already reduced, as in a high-flying jet aircraft, heavy smokers may become particularly sensitive to the effects of carbon monoxide and develop symptoms of poisoning. Moreover, even in the absence of obvious effects, CO has a definite action on the wall of the blood-vessels, making them more permeable than normal. This probably allows more fatty substances to pass from the bloodstream into the wall of the blood-vessel, another action which may predispose smokers to develop atheroma (p. 300).

WHY PEOPLE SMOKE

One in twenty of ten- and eleven-year-old children have already started smoking. Most smokers, however, start as adolescents, girls usually later than boys. Only 15 per cent of adolescents who have smoked more than one cigarette avoid becoming permanent smokers, while only 15 per cent of regular smokers manage to give the habit up before the age of sixty. At first, adolescents smoke for psychological reasons: they think it makes them look tough and grown up, and their parents and friends do not discourage them. Another reason for starting smoking may be to compensate for poor achievement: boys who smoke regularly do not do as well at schoolwork or games as non-smokers.

Having started, people tend to go on smoking for one of three main reasons: continuing social ones (such as in company); 'indulgence' smoking for pleasure, often after meals, with a drink or together with activities such as reading or watching television; or to satisfy 'inner need' – such as for calm, stimulation or addiction. Several facts suggest that many smokers are mildly habituated to nicotine in cigarette smoke. Only 2 per cent of smokers do not smoke regularly, while only 9 per cent of men and 19 per cent of women do not inhale. Heavy smokers inhale more than light ones and young smokers more than older ones. Experiments in which regular smokers performed various tasks while they were smoking low- or high-nicotine cigarettes showed that they adjusted their puffing frequency to obtain a constant dose of nicotine. Three out of every four smokers wish to stop the habit, but only one of them succeeds. On stopping smoking some people develop mild physical withdrawal symptoms (such as sleep disturbances, sweating and a fall in pulse rate and blood pressure); these effects are reversed by an injection of pure nicotine.

Cigarette smokers have been said to differ from non-smokers in personality, being more extroverted and less rigid, while pipe smokers have been claimed to be more introverted than either cigarette smokers or non-smokers. If such differences exist, they are very small, and there is no evidence that people with definite psychiatric illness are more likely to smoke more.

DEATH STATISTICS

At all ages smokers have a higher death rate than non-smokers. This difference is mostly small for pipe or cigar smokers but appreciable for cigarette smokers and is directly related to the number of cigarettes smoked every day, particularly in younger men. Studying the mortality rate over a twelve-year period in almost 41,000 British doctors whose smoking habits were known, Doll and Hill showed that this was 19 per cent higher among smokers and 28 per cent higher among cigarette smokers; even so, in pure pipe or cigar smokers the increase was only 1 per cent. The death rate increased progressively so that in people who smoked twenty-five cigarettes a day it was 63 per cent above that in life-long non-smokers. Similarly, research in the USA showed that in non-smokers aged between thirty-five and forty-four the annual death rate was 2·1 per 1,000, compared with that in those smoking over forty cigarettes a day of 5·5. In men aged between sixty-five and seventy-four the death rates per 1,000 were thirty-one and fifty-six for non-smokers and smokers, respectively.

From these figures it has been calculated that probably over 35,000 deaths a year in people between thirty-five and sixty-four are associated with smoking – and that at least 27,500 of these are directly due to the habit. Two in every five heavy cigarette smokers are likely to die before their sixty-fifth birthday, double the proportion of life-long non-smokers. These last figures are based on reports which have shown that cigarette smoking is an important fact in three major diseases of adults: lung cancer, chronic bronchitis and emphysema, and coronary heart disease. In addition we now know that cigarette smoking during pregnancy increases the mortality rate in the embryo and young baby by 28 per cent, representing the deaths of 1,500 babies a year in Great Britain.

LUNG CANCER

There had been two or three anecdotal accounts of a possible link between cancer of the lung and tobacco smoking, but the first statistical proof was provided in 1950 by Bradford Hill and Doll. They had started a large-scale inquiry in 1947 by interviewing four groups of patients from twenty London hospitals with cancer of the lung, stomach and large bowel, as well as a control group of patients who did not have cancer but were matched individually for age and sex with the lung cancer patients. All patients were asked for full details of their smoking habits over their whole lives, a smoker being defined as somebody who had smoked at least one cigarette a day for a year.

Bradford Hill and Doll showed that the vast majority of men with lung cancer had smoked at some time in their lives. Only two out of 649 patients (0·3 per cent) were non-smokers compared with twenty-seven non-smokers out of 649 non-cancer control patients (4·2 per cent), and the trend was similar for women, in whom at that time smoking was much less common. The same difference was found in comparing smoking habits of the patients with lung cancer with those of patients with other types of cancer added to those in the control group. Moreover, the risk of lung cancer was greater in heavy smokers than in light ones, and seemed to vary in proportion to the amount smoked. Cigarette smoking was much more closely related to lung cancer than pipe smoking, but no distinct association was found with inhaling. Similar results were reported at the same time from the USA by Wynder and Graham.

All this research had started from the observation of a meteoric rise in lung cancer deaths, which per million men in England and Wales had been ten in 1900, thirteen in 1910, seventeen in 1920, fifty-five in 1930, 187 in 1940 and 484 in 1950; the corresponding figures for women were seven, nine, ten, twenty-one, forty-nine and eighty-eight. By 1955 the death rate was double that only ten years earlier, and was causing one in eighteen of all deaths in men (though only one in 103 deaths in women). Today in Britain lung cancer is the commonest lethal cancer in men.

Publicizing these facts two years after Bradford Hill and Doll's report, a statement by the British Medical Research Council advised the government that a major part of this increase was associated with cigarette smoking. It emphasized that no fewer than nineteen inquiries had shown a definite link between lung cancer and smoking, and that the risk increased with the amount smoked. The risk was linked with two of the three types of cancer ('squamous' and 'oat-cell') but not with the adenocarcinomatous variety.

The drawback to accepting these results as proof of the link was that all these inquiries had been retrospective. In other words, they had compared the smoking habits of patients with lung cancer with those of healthy people or those with some illness probably unrelated to smoking, or the incidence of lung cancer in smokers with that in non-smokers. But in 1951 Bradford Hill and Doll started another type of study – a prospective investigation, to record the smoking habits of a given population at a given time and then to follow the group to see what its members died from.

They chose to study how the smoking habits of doctors changed over a particular period and to compare this and the death rates from various conditions with the rest of the population. In October 1951 they sent a questionnaire to all British doctors asking them about their smoking habits, and repeated this for men in 1957 and 1966 and for women in 1961. They obtained details of the cause of death of those doctors who died during the three separate periods from death certificates and checked these in various ways.

Between 1951 and 1966 the proportion of male doctors who were non-smokers rose from 34 per cent to 51 per cent while that of cigarette smokers fell from 43 per cent to 21 per cent. For men in the whole population, over the same period the proportions remained more or less unaltered, at 30 per cent and 40 per cent respectively. In doctors the over-all death rate from disease considered to be related to smoking in Bradford Hill and Doll's first report stayed much the same, at about 7·40 per 1,000 annually; in the general population it increased from 8·43 in 1954–7 to 10·8 in 1962–5. For lung-cancer deaths the differences between the two groups were particularly striking: in doctors the rate fell by 25 per cent, while in the general population it increased by 26 per cent. Moreover, if men aged only thirty-five to sixty-four were considered (in whom the diagnosis was virtually bound to be certain) the differences showed exactly the same trend: a decline of 38 per cent for cancer of the lung in male doctors compared with an increase of 7 per cent for the whole population.

The results of this study probably represent the most convincing evidence of the link between smoking and lung cancer, as well as the fact that stopping immediately lessens the risk. In particular, they refute some of the arguments that the dramatic rise in lung-cancer figures has been due to hereditary predisposition to develop the disease in response to cigarette smoking or to air pollution, such as diesel fumes. Certainly in smokers the incidence of lung cancer is higher in urban compared with rural areas, and a similar additive effect is seen in some industries, lung cancer being commoner in those involving chromate, asbestos, nickel and tar. Nevertheless, air pollution is diminishing rather than increasing; diesel fumes do not contain high levels of known cancer-producing substances; the dramatic rise in lung cancer began before these fumes became very prevalent; non-smokers exposed to traffic fumes, such as policemen on point duty, do not have a higher incidence of lung cancer than those not so exposed; and research in countries where there is no pollution at all (such as Rhodesia and the Channel Isles) has emphasized the straight link between the number of cigarettes smoked and the risk of lung cancer.

Recent figures for lung cancer are also answering another objection – that the much lower incidence in women smokers does not parallel their cigarette consumption. So far men have been five times as likely to develop lung cancer as women, but they smoke only twice as much. But women started to smoke heavily comparatively recently; on average, they begin the habit later than boys, inhale less and tend to smoke milder cigarettes. The increase in their death rate from lung cancer is now occurring more rapidly than that in men, and this supports the generally accepted thesis that a lag period of at least twenty years is necessary for the development of most cancers related to an outside cause.

Another objection to the simple idea of cause and effect is that in only a few experiments have research workers produced lung cancer in animals by exposing them to an atmosphere of tobacco smoke – although dogs taught to inhale did develop the disease. But laboratory animals do not always react to substances in the same way as man; conversely, for instance, some substances will cause cancer in them which seem to be harmless in humans (p. 73). Not only does tar contain several known cancer-producing agents, but it also produces skin tumours in several different animal species. Finally microscopical examination of the air passages from some smokers shows important differences from those of non-smokers: an absence of cilia and changes in the cells on the surface suggesting precancer. These changes are greater in heavy smokers compared with light ones and tend to regress in those who give up smoking.

CHRONIC BRONCHITIS AND EMPHYSEMA

Chronic bronchitis is a serious disease of the air passages in which these produce too much mucus (the slime that normally coats and lubricates them). The mucus causes persistent cough and phlegm, an increased tendency to chest infections (particularly in the winter) and gradual impairment of lung efficiency. In emphysema, which is often associated with a long history of chronic bronchitis, many of the tiny air sacs of the lungs are destroyed: again, this results in impaired lung efficiency and it may also eventually seriously strain the heart.

In Britain chronic bronchitis and emphysema are particularly common, killing 30,000 people every year, and are known as the 'English disease'. The causes (p. 189) are complex. Up to adolescence air pollution and social class are important associated factors, but by the age of twenty cigarette smoking is the dominant influence. Among twenty-year-olds winter cough by day or night is more than twice as common in smokers as in non-smokers. In adults this is even more obvious: 91 per cent of a group of 300 chronic bronchitics were found to be smokers, compared with 79 per cent of 300 healthy controls matched for age, sex and social class. Lung function in apparently healthy people is less efficient in smokers compared with non-smokers. Combining the results of seven separate studies, the American Surgeon General reported that smokers died six times as frequently from bronchitis as would have been expected. In the group of British doctors studied by Bradford Hill and Doll the death rate from bronchitis in those smoking over twenty-five cigarettes a day was more than twenty times that in non-smokers. Research has also shown that the risk is directly proportional to the amount smoked; is less in non-inhalers, smokers of filter-tipped cigarettes, and pipe smokers; and generally diminishes in people who give up smoking.

Chronic bronchitis is also linked with cancer of the lung. This type of cancer is commoner in people with chronic bronchitis, irrespective of age and the amount of tobacco smoked. Smokers with a cough have double the incidence of cancer as those without – although only half of all lung cancer develops in patients with a cough.

Although we still do not know exactly how chronic bronchitis evolves, the likely sequence seems to be that the irritants in the cigarette smoke stimulate the lining of the air passages to produce more mucus; but the mucus is not removed in the usual way because the cilia have been either damaged or destroyed by smoking. Instead, it is coughed up as phlegm during the traditional 'smoker's cough' – which is present even in young people. This stage is known as 'simple bronchitis'; in the next, 'recurrent infective bronchitis', the mucus becomes infected by bacteria, giving rise to episodes of acute illness with fever and phlegm discoloured by pus; it is at this stage that factors such as air pollution, social class and occupation play an important additional part. In the final stage, 'chronic obstructive bronchitis', the air passages become choked with infected mucus and the air sacs are destroyed, leading to the formation of large air cysts in the lungs with a diminution in their ability to take up oxygen and dispose of carbon dioxide.

DISEASES OF THE HEART AND BLOOD-VESSELS

Coronary heart disease (CHD; p. 44) is now the commonest cause of death in Britain, being responsible for 100,000 deaths a year, 31,000 in men under the age of sixty-five. Smoking is one of the important features known to predispose towards the development of CHD, ranking in importance with high blood-pressure and a raised serum cholesterol level. Under the age of fifty-five coronary attacks are three times as common in moderate smokers (fifteen cigarettes a day) as in non-smokers, and the risk of sudden death is five times as great. After sixty-five the differential risk decreases, being about one and a half times commoner in smokers. In those who have recovered from one coronary attack, giving up smoking is the only factor statistically known to reduce the risk of another one. Again, there is a direct link with the number of cigarettes smoked as well as inhalation, and a much diminished risk with pipe and cigar smoking. For example, men aged forty to forty-nine who smoke forty cigarettes a day have five times the risk of dying from CHD as non-smokers. Stopping smoking also reduces the risk: in Bradford Hill and Doll's group of doctors the death rates from heart disease fell by 6 per cent, whereas at the same time in the general population they rose by 9 per cent.

Atheromatous disease of the arteries elsewhere in the body is also related to smoking. Atheroma in the aorta is more extensive in smokers compared with non-smokers, while 95 per cent of patients with arterial disease are smokers. In a group of patients treated by grafts for arterial disease in the legs, one fifth of the grafts failed in patients who continued to smoke after operation, compared with no failures in patients who gave up smoking.

We still know comparatively little about how smoking produces these effects on the arteries and the heart. The action of nicotine in making platelets more sticky may be important in causing atheroma. In established atheroma of the coronary arteries nicotine may increase the work done by the heart and raise the amount of oxygen it uses without raising the blood-flow in the arteries; possibly this leads to dangerous irregularities of heart rhythm. Recent research, however, has focused attention on the possible important role of CO. A combined Danish–British study found that people aged thirty to sixty-nine with a blood-CO level of 5 per cent or over were twenty-one times as likely to be affected by arteriosclerosis (coronary heart disease and narrowing of the arteries supplying the legs) as people of the same age and smoking habits but with a level of under 3 per cent. CO is known to damage the wall of blood-vessels, but an equally important action may be to deprive the heart of much-needed oxygen, by combining with some of the haemoglobin in the red blood cells.

An estimated 10,000 deaths a year from CHD in people in England and Wales under sixty-five would not occur if they stopped smoking cigarettes, while numerically the importance of deaths from CHD at all ages outweighs those due to lung cancer. Professor D. D. Reid of the London School of Hygiene has calculated that of every 100 deaths attributable to heavy smoking about sixteen may be due to lung cancer, but no fewer than fifty may result from CHD. Certainly, American projects for trying to cut down CHD deaths in people identified as being especially coronary-prone have found that other preventive measures are of limited value unless the person gives up smoking.

SMOKING AND PREGNANCY

The fourth known major aspect of tobacco smoking is its effect on the unborn baby. The British Perinatal Mortality Survey found that, compared with non-smokers, women who smoke during pregnancy have a doubled incidence of miscarriage, a 30 per cent higher stillbirth rate, and a 26 per cent higher death rate among their new-born babies, who are smaller at birth, weighing an average of 150–250 grammes less. All these effects have led to an estimate that if no mother in Britain smoked after the fourth month of pregnancy about 1,500 more babies would survive every year. Even at seven and eleven years of age on average these children are still probably undersized and show some educational retardation.

Most of these effects are related to the smaller size of the baby, since the death rate rises fairly steeply in those weighing under 2·5 kg. at birth. The reduction in size results from the diminished supply of oxygen to the foetus during pregnancy, and is much the same as that seen in babies born to mothers living at high altitudes, compared with those born to mothers living at sea-level. Again, in mothers who smoke the higher levels of CO in the bloodstream are almost certainly responsible for depriving the foetus of some of its oxygen supply.

OTHER RISKS

Two other types of cancer of the air passages are probably related to tobacco. The first type, of the passages in the nose, occurs in snuff-takers and is presumably due to direct irritation of the lining of the nose by the snuff. The second type, of the larynx, is probably commoner in smokers compared with non-smokers, and in heavy smokers compared with lighter ones. Only 13 per cent of one series of patients with laryngeal cancer were non-smokers, compared with 41 per cent of controls. Even so, there are still difficulties in regarding this association as proved: cancer of the larynx is rare and its incidence has not increased over the last seventy years. This discrepancy could be because laryngeal cancer is caused by several factors, some of which have disappeared in the last few years; because it is difficult to classify tumours in this part of the body; or because the supposed link does not in fact exist.

Smoking may also contribute to the development of tuberculosis in middle or later life: almost 88 per cent of men patients were smokers or had smoked fewer than ten cigarettes a day, compared with 79 per cent of controls – while 50 per cent had smoked twenty cigarettes a day or more compared with 43 per cent of controls. Deaths from pulmonary tuberculosis are also commoner in smokers compared with non-smokers, and smoking probably causes healed or quiescent tuberculous lung disease to break down.

Both gastric and duodenal ulcers are commoner in smokers (particularly gastric ulcers) and are more frequent in heavy compared with light smokers and in those who smoke cigarettes rather than pipes or cigars. Research has shown that during smoking the contents of the first part of the duodenum can return past the pyloric valve back into the stomach. This action, which does not occur in non-smoking healthy people, leads to bile entering the stomach and this can probably damage its lining and lead to ulceration. Smoking has a similar action on another valve in the digestive system – that separating the oesophagus, or gullet, from the stomach. This action may explain the commonness in smokers of heartburn, due to the acid stomach contents passing into the lower part of the oesophagus. Continuing to smoke cigarettes delays the healing of ulcers induced by medical treatment, while the death rate from both types of ulcer is six times as high in smokers as in non-smokers. Even so, the geographical distribution of the death rate from ulcers is quite different from the pattern of tobacco smoking, and probably the link comes about because of this delay in ulcer healing – which increases the risk of serious complications.

Two other conditions strongly associated with smoking are cirrhosis of the liver and alcoholism (p. 212), which are between 1·3 and four times as common in smokers as non-smokers. This is probably because heavy drinkers are also heavy smokers.

Several reports have suggested that cancer of the kidney is linked with smoking, but further research is needed to confirm this. Undoubtedly, however, cancer of the urinary bladder is commoner in smokers and the association is stronger in heavy compared with light smokers. The risk also seems to exist for pipe and cigar smokers. Respectively men and women cigarette smokers are 1·89 and 2·0 times as likely to develop bladder cancer as non-smokers, and about 39 per cent and 29 per cent of all cases are probably related to smoking. It has also been claimed that the outlook is worse in treated patients who continue to smoke compared with that in those who give it up. There is also a strong link between death rates from lung cancer and bladder cancer for twenty countries, confirming that the association of the latter with smoking is real; but the mechanism of this action on the bladder remains unknown.

DIFFERENTIAL RISKS

Pipe and cigar smokers seem to run a risk only a little higher than non-smokers, although most surveys have contained too few people in these groups for full statistical analysis. The reasons for this difference are not clear, since pipe and cigar smoke contain more nicotine and tar and much the same amount of irritants and carbon monoxide. Possible differences include chemical make-up — cigarette smoke is acid, whereas pipe and cigar smoke are alkaline — and the amount inhaled: nicotine in alkaline smoke is readily absorbed from the membranes lining the mouth, whereas nicotine in acid smoke is not and needs to be drawn into the lungs. Cigarette smokers who switch to another form of smoking tend to go on inhaling so that their blood-CO levels, for instance, stay in the zone associated with a greatly increased risk of CHD. A careful study of these 'secondary' pipe or cigar smokers (if a large enough group can be found) might answer the questions about the role of inhaling.

In their original report Bradford Hill and Doll said that they could find no conclusive difference between the risks run by cigarette smokers who inhaled and those who did not. But later research has shown that the former, who are in the majority, do have an increased risk of lung cancer, bronchitis and heart disease, and that the risks are less in people who smoke filter cigarettes and in those who do not smoke cigarettes right down to a very short butt (such as women and the inhabitants of the USA). Tar tends to condense in the cooler part of the cigarette nearer to the smoker's mouth, so that discarding a relatively long butt may discard a disproportionate amount of dangerous tar.

Another controversy has concerned whether some types of

cigarettes are less likely to produce cancer than others. Tobacco (for pipes, cigars and cigarettes) is prepared in two main ways – air-curing and flue-curing. Air-curing takes about three months and involves drying the tobacco in special barns without heat. Flue-curing takes only six days and involves drying the tobacco in similar barns but using artificial heat at a temperature of about 80°C. In air-cured tobacco the sugar content is low, because it has been destroyed during curing by the action of enzymes (chemical catalysts). In flue-cured tobacco, however, the sugar content is considerable (25 per cent or more) because the high curing temperature destroys the enzymes.

In Britain most cigarette tobacco is flue-cured, whereas in some other countries it is air-cured, or a mixture of the two types; cigar and some pipe tobaccos are air-cured. The late Professor Richard Passey suggested that one of the reasons that lung cancer had become so common, and that the risks of smoking the same amount of tobacco in cigars were so much less than in cigarettes, was the difference in the sugar content of the tobaccos. He and a research team tested both types of tobacco and claimed that the smoke of the flue-cured variety was more dangerous to man and animals: it greatly shortened the life of rats and damaged their air passages, whereas the smoke of air-cured tobacco was relatively harmless. Even so, experts have challenged these conclusions, particularly because the experiments were inadequately controlled and the rats died of inflammation of the lungs and air passages rather than of cancer.

Furthermore, other researchers have shown that tars from the two types of tobacco painted on the skin of mice produce the same number of tumours. Another approach to this problem, by comparing death rates from lung cancer in different countries, is fraught with difficulties – for example, in comparing only France and England. In the former total tobacco consumption per head is still less than in the latter; thirty years ago Frenchmen smoked between a third and a half of the cigarettes they do today; and even now only half of the French smoking population inhale, compared with 80–90 per cent of Englishmen.

All this means that we cannot say that cigarette smokers run a lesser risk of lung cancer if they switch to air-cured tobacco. There have been two other approaches to finding a 'safer' cigarette: to classify individual cigarettes by their content of nicotine and tar, and to develop tobacco substitutes. In Britain the Health Departments have published a 'league table' giving the tar and nicotine yields of 101 different brands of cigarette, with Capstan Full Strength (tar 38 mg., nicotine 3·2 mg.) and Silk Cut Extra Mild (tar 4 mg., nicotine 0·3 mg.) occupying the top and bottom places, respectively. Smokers who cannot give up have been recommended to switch to one with a low content of both (in general a low-nicotine cigarette tends to be a low-tar one as well). Nevertheless, addicted smokers adjust their smoking habits to obtain a constant nicotine intake, and are often unwilling to switch to a very-low-nicotine cigarette. The present league table also ignores the third major harmful component of cigarette smoke: CO. Dr Michael Hamilton Russell, a psychiatrist at London's Maudsley Hospital who has carried out much research into smoking addiction, has shown that cigarettes vary widely in their CO content, and that switching to either the brand at the top or at the bottom of the league table might lower CO levels – in the former case because the cigarette contains so much nicotine that people smoke less, and in the latter because the CO content is low anyway. So the safest cigarette for the addicted smoker who inhales might be one with a low tar and CO level, but with a high nicotine content. At present such a cigarette seems not to exist, but eventually manufacturers should be able to produce one. In the meantime the government should add CO yields to its cigarette league table.

Objections also apply to the introduction of smoking substitutes. Long-term tests are needed to ensure that no new hazards are being introduced, since burning any substance produces CO as well as substances able to cause cancer.

There also remains the difficulty of applying the results of laboratory tests in animals to recommendations for smokers. The addicted smoker, moreover, seems unlikely to switch to a product which does not give him the amount of nicotine he 'needs'. If the tobacco substitute is mixed with an equal amount of ordinary tobacco the smoker may merely smoke twice as many of the new cigarettes, thereby increasing his intake of CO and tar. At present research is concentrating on developing NSP (New Smoking Product), prepared from wood cellulose, which produces only one quarter of the tar of cigarettes. Possibly this could be introduced into conventional cigarettes in gradually increasing amounts. All these considerations have led the British government to set up a special medical committee (the Hunter Committee) to advise manufacturers confidentially about the scientific aspects of any new products.

RISKS OF SMOKING TO NON-SMOKERS

Although official reports have pressed for limiting smoking in places of entertainment and on public transport, to try to cut down the opportunities for smokers, there has been little mention of any risk to the non-smoker from other people's tobacco smoke. To some extent this was understandable for although a few people are truly allergic to tobacco smoke – developing asthma if they are exposed to it – most non-smokers find it only a disagreeable nuisance, and the early results of research showed that one had to inhale cigarette smoke regularly to absorb appreciable quantities of nicotine and tar. But the situation has probably changed since the more recent studies focused attention on the importance of CO in human illness, particularly diseases of the heart and blood-vessels. In another project Dr Hamilton Russell and his colleagues studied twelve non-smoking volunteers who spent about an hour and a quarter in a smoke-filled room ($15 \times 12 \times 8$ ft; the smoke being produced from a total of eighty cigarettes and two cigars). Blood-CO levels rose by an average of 1 per cent – much the same as if they had smoked and inhaled one cigarette.

In another experiment, by a German doctor, the smoking of ten cigarettes over an hour in a closed car caused the blood-CO level in two non-smokers to rise from 2 per cent to 5 per cent. Scientists have now shown that levels of 3 per cent and over may have subtle effects on perception, making it more difficult to discriminate between small differences in light intensity and impairing the sense of time. Research into other aspects of passively absorbed tobacco smoke is still going on.

ECONOMIC ASPECTS

Many politicians have claimed that, apart from any other consideration, the amount of tax received from tobacco every year would make it impossible to abolish cigarette smoking. Yet large though the revenue is (£1,275 million in 1974), several other factors have to be put on the other side of the balance sheet. No fewer than 8,500 hospital beds are occupied as a result of cigarette smoking, at an annual cost of £25 million. Compared with non-smokers, smokers are known to be excessive users of the National Health Service; some of the most expensive drugs prescribed in the Service are antibiotics, used in treating bronchitis among other illnesses. Moreover, statistics show that all respiratory disease accounted for 21·1 per cent of all working days lost in 1970–71 (including about 33 million days lost from acute bronchitis alone) while diseases of the circulatory system accounted for another 14·0 per cent.

If everybody stopped cigarette smoking it would save an estimated minimum of 35,000 lives a year, while if the public gave up on the same scale as doctors some 8,000 lives would be saved a year. These 35,000 premature deaths every year from lung cancer, bronchitis and CHD entail a loss to the community of £270 million in lost production and earnings together with the need to pay widow's pensions. Finally, official studies in both the USA and Canada have concluded that in these countries abolishing cigarette smoking would produce greater savings in health care costs, lost production and pensions than losses from revenue to the taxman.

GIVING IT UP

About half of all smokers wish to give up the habit, but the variety of methods used for this – hypnotism, aversion therapy, smoking clinics and group therapy – testify partly to the addictive feature of smoking and partly to the social pressures which suggest that it is a normal, acceptable practice. Most people who want to give up mention minor upsets to their health, such as frequent colds and 'poor wind', rather than worry over serious conditions such as lung cancer. The next most frequent reason is to save money. The results of formal anti-smoking measures such as clinics are disappointing: the success rate is 30–40 per cent immediately and 12–30 per cent at the end of the year – much the same as the spontaneous discontinuance rate of 20–30 per cent in the untreated population. For well-motivated highly addicted people who want to give up smoking, aversion therapy may be useful, but for the average person firm advice from a doctor to abandon smoking is as likely to be successful as any more complicated treatment; the more motivated a person is the more likely he is to be successful. More men in the upper social classes (who are more likely to appreciate that the serious risks of smoking are real) have given up smoking than those in the lower social classes.

Giving up smoking is often easier for the patient with an obvious motive such as a smoking-linked disease, for example bronchitis or coronary heart disease, than for the healthy, often younger, person – who is unlikely to be influenced by the doctor pointing out that it is an expensive habit impairing taste and causing him to smell unsavoury to his non-smoking friends. Those who want to stop but find it difficult should find a sympathetic doctor who is keen on helping him and believes that the habit can be abandoned, given a well-planned campaign. This aims at stopping smoking completely within a short time, certainly within a month. For those who cannot stop immediately some experts recommend first switching to a low-tar brand, recording every cigarette smoked, progressively omitting the cigarette that gives the most pleasure, and smoking the first cigarette an hour later each day. One of the most difficult problems is the ex-smoker who relapses under stress: not uncommonly one sees people faced with a difficult situation thrust their hands into a jacket pocket for a cigarette, though they have not smoked for twenty years. Some ex-smokers also say that even if they had one after-dinner cigar they would be back smoking cigarettes again, so powerful is the hold on them. The doctor can help his patients by encouragement in the early days of abstinence from smoking, while some people are helped by group therapy – similar to Weight-Watchers Clubs. There is no evidence, however, that medicinal drugs, chewing sweets or gum helps much in the difficult cases.

Anti-smoking campaigns are most likely to be effective in those who have never started. Adults who have tried and failed to stop smoking should at very least try to discourage children and teenagers from experimenting with cigarettes; experts believe that a child may be addicted after smoking as few as five to ten cigarettes.

To give up smoking successfully a clean break seems the best practice. In spite of popular belief, only 14 per cent of people find giving up very difficult, although some heavy smokers complain of increased irritability and restlessness in the first few weeks. One major health hazard – obesity – is inversely related to smoking: non-smokers weigh more than smokers and smokers who give up smoking put on weight. Research in a group of Welsh steel-workers showed that in smokers weight tended to level off after the age of thirty-five, but in non-smokers it increased until about fifty. On average non-smokers weighed 13 lb. more than smokers, but ex-smokers took over eight years to gain this amount of weight after giving up the habit. From the results of this survey it is difficult to assess the relative risks of smoking and obesity, for both the smokers and non-smokers were considerably overweight – by about 15 lb. and 30 lb., respectively – and this may not be a feature of other social classes or occupations, such as businessmen. However, the authors of the Welsh report comment that any suggestion that to be 10 lb. overweight carries a greater health risk than smoking twenty-five cigarettes a day is almost certainly untrue.

Finally, the doctors in Bradford Hill and Doll's study who gave up smoking reported more advantages than disadvantages; only 5 per cent were more tense or irritable, compared with 10 per cent of those who were still smoking, while 24 per cent said they were more energetic, compared with 3 per cent of the smokers. All this makes it difficult for many doctors to maintain their objectivity. They naturally wonder why so many people continue with such a dangerous habit, and, if this chapter has seemed to present an excessively gloomy picture, it is as well to end it with a quotation from Bradford Hill and Doll's report of the benefits obtained by the doctors who gave up smoking. 'One of the striking characteristics of British mortality in the last half-century has been the lack of improvement in the death rate of men in their middle life. In cigarette smoking may lie one prominent cause.'

Chapter 13

SEX

'MAKING love is a mental disease which wastes time and energy' – or so the Chinese people were told during the wave of puritanism during the Cultural Revolution in 1969. However, few human activities are less influenced by rational argument than sexual relationships. Perhaps it is as well, therefore, that there is no convincing medical evidence that sexual activity is either strikingly good or bad for the health; instead there is a balance sheet of hazards and advantages which must be assessed by each individual in the light of his inclinations.

Sexual activity does affect susceptibility to disease and expectation of life, but at present the evidence is mainly indirect. Differences in mortality associated with sexual activity are more obvious in women, since the Registrar General distinguishes between married and single women but not between married and single men. The annual statistics based on death certificates show convincingly that at all ages after twenty single women have a higher mortality rate than married – but both are lower than the rate for men. In part the difference between single and married women may be explained by the lower chances of marriage for a woman who is handicapped by poor health, but this cannot explain the continuing difference in later years. Child-bearing still has a mortality, and married women are more likely to develop cancer of the cervix; but cancer of the breast and uterus are more common in women who have not borne children. However, the differences in mortality seen in conditions such as heart disease and stroke are still unexplained. There seems some non-specific contentment factor that goes with marriage – and which could explain the perhaps apocryphal longevity of Church of England clergy-

257

men compared with their Roman Catholic counterparts.

For many middle-aged men and women sexual intercourse is their most physically demanding activity. If either partner is known to have heart disease or raised blood pressure there may be some reasonable apprehension that intercourse could precipitate a heart attack or a stroke. For a man a single act of intercourse may require as much physical effort as fifteen to twenty press-ups (see p. 105), but such energetic love-making is not essential; in practice the amount of physical effort expended can be varied to suit the inclinations of the couple. The usual medical advice given to someone who has had a coronary thrombosis is that normal sexual activity may be resumed after about three months. At that stage sexual intercourse is no more likely to blow a fuse than coping with constipation or eating a large Sunday lunch. Heart patients who get angina – chest pain brought on by exertion – generally take a nitroglycerine tablet before climbing a flight of stairs or walking up a hill, and it is just as sensible to take a tablet before sex. In general, however, physicians nowadays recommend their patients with cardiovascular disease to take regular physical exercise, and sexual intercourse is an excellent way to achieve this.

Until this century, the great hazards of sexual activity were pregnancy and venereal disease. Death in childbirth happened to the rich and famous – Princess Charlotte, Mrs Beeton – and repeated confinements multiplied the risks, so that Queen Victoria could count herself fortunate to have survived eleven pregnancies.

Nowadays death associated with pregnancy is rare, but it may and does occur. Each year nearly 100 women die in childbirth or of complications of pregnancy; and another fifty die from miscarriage or abortion. This is the yardstick against which the risks of modern contraceptive methods must be measured, for a woman who is sexually active for twenty to thirty-five years might otherwise expect to become pregnant again on average seven months after the birth of each baby. At present in Britain the risk of death for a woman who becomes pregnant is about twenty deaths for every 100,000 births. Complications of childbirth itself account for some half of these deaths, and the others are made up of deaths from miscarriage and illness during pregnancy. The risk rises with age, and is about two and a half times greater at forty than at twenty. Some deaths occur in high-risk patients – women with heart or kidney disease who are prepared to risk pregnancy despite the advice given by their doctors. Others are essentially accidents – the birth is not straightforward, an anaesthetic has to be given, and possibly an operation performed: all these proceedings carry a small but unavoidable risk that the heart will stop or some other disaster occur. Deaths associated with childbirth are unique in one way: every one is investigated by a confidential inquiry organized by the Department of Health, and the results of these inquiries are regularly published. In fact British mortality figures have fallen from sixty-seven per 100,000 in 1952 to less than twenty per 100,000 in 1973, and are as good as any in the world.

ABORTION

If the pregnancy is unwanted a woman may have it terminated if there are legal grounds – defined by the Abortion Act 1967 as reasonable grounds for believing either that the child would be abnormal or that the continuance of the pregnancy would involve greater risk than termination itself to the life or health of the woman or to her existing children. In deciding the extent of the risk a doctor has to take account of the actual and foreseeable environment. Since the introduction of the Act in 1968 the number of terminations done has settled at about 100,000 each year (not counting women who come to Britain solely to arrange an abortion), and some authorities argue that this figure – one abortion for every eight completed pregnancies – is no higher than the one for illegal abortions before 1968.

Experience with abortions since the change in the law in 1967 has shown that the risks of the operation are much higher later in pregnancy. In 1971 Professor Sir John Stallworthy analysed the results of over 1,000 terminations of pregnancy in Oxford hospitals. He found that serious complications such as postoperative bleeding, infection and damage to the uterus were between two and eight times as common when the pregnancy had lasted longer than ten weeks. A similar ratio is found for deaths due to abortion, though the numbers are small. Nevertheless, statistics published by the Department of Health show that each year about 25 per cent of all legal terminations of pregnancy are done later than thirteen weeks' gestation – an indication of the delays that occur between a woman becoming aware of her pregnancy and termination being arranged.

What of the long-term consequences of abortion? Few subjects have provoked such bitter and emotional argument within the medical profession. Undoubtedly a woman who has an abortion incurs some risk of sub-fertility – she may not be able to become pregnant again – and if she does become pregnant she runs an increased risk of a miscarriage, complications during pregnancy and premature labour. The dispute is about how to measure these risks. They can be assessed only by doctors keeping careful and complete records of the subsequent medical history of every woman who has an abortion for at least five years. Most of the statistics quoted refer to abortions done in Eastern Europe and Japan in the 1950s and 1960s; and these may be criticized as 'unreliable' by those who do not like them. Furthermore, techniques have changed rapidly in the last year or two, and many doctors believe that 'lunchtime abortions', in which a thin tube is used to empty the uterus by suction, carry a negligible risk of late complications. Others put the risk of long-term ill-effects as high as 30 per cent.

In 1973 the Foundation for Education and Research in Childbearing published a long analysis by Dr Margaret and

Dr Arthur Wynn of the consequences of induced abortion to children born subsequently. They reviewed statistics from all over the world and claimed that after an abortion there was a 2–5 per cent risk that the woman would be unable ever again to become pregnant. If she did become pregnant the Wynn report suggested that the risk of the baby being born prematurely was increased by 40 per cent and that of its dying shortly after birth was increased by 50 per cent. The report put the risk of ectopic pregnancy (in which the fertilized egg starts its development outside the uterus) at two to three times normal. Estimates of the effect of abortion on subsequent general health are more difficult, since there are fewer clear-cut criteria; but there is no doubt that the operation does increase the risk of irregular menstruation and chronic inflammation of the uterus.

Perhaps a combination of further improvements in technique and termination earlier in pregnancy will cut the rate of complications in future; but they will never be eliminated any more than complications of childbirth. Based on a middle-of-the-road assessment of risks, abortion carried out early in pregnancy is less dangerous to a woman's health than allowing the pregnancy to continue normally; but there is the enormous and important difference that most women will accept the small element of risk in having a baby but will not so readily accept the risks of abortion.

RELIABILITY OF CONTRACEPTIVES

So long as pregnancy remains a risky business, the possible health hazards of different contraceptive methods should be measured against the risks of unintentional pregnancy ending either in abortion or in childbirth. Mechanical methods such as the sheath or diaphragm carry no direct risk to health; but the failure rate is relatively high. The Family Planning Association estimate of the failure rates of current methods of contraception are shown in the table:

	Pregnancy/100 women-years' exposure
Douche	40·8
Rhythm	38·5
Withdrawal	16·8
Diaphragm	14·4
Condom	13·8

Even the most reliable of these methods, the condom, may be expected to result in an unwanted pregnancy after about eight years, and the other methods are even less trustworthy. Of course, many unwanted pregnancies lead to the birth of a child that is loved as well as any of his planned brothers or sisters; but there is a risk to the health or life of the mother from the 'normal' process of pregnancy.

THE PILL

The introduction of contraceptive pills in the 1960s represented a major revolution in family planning; for the first time a method of birth control was available that could be totally effective and need not interfere with the spontaneity of sexual intercourse. Unfortunately as experience with the use of contraceptive pills accumulated it became clear that the powerful synthetic hormones they contained had a wide range of unwanted effects.

Almost all oral contraceptives contain a mixture of two sex hormones, oestrogen and progestogen. The synthetic compounds used are very similar to the natural hormones produced by the ovary during the usual menstrual cycle, and their presence in the blood blocks the normal monthly process of ovulation. These 'combined' pills have a multiple contraceptive action: the suppression of ovulation stops the release of any eggs into the uterus; they change the lining of the uterus so that it can no longer nourish an egg if one were fertilized; and they change the consistency of the mucus at the lower end of the womb so that sperm cannot penetrate it. This triple action is the basis of the remarkable reliability of

oral contraception, since pregnancy is most unlikely to result
if a woman forgets one or two doses in a monthly cycle.

Unfortunately this interference with the normal hormonal balance may lead to unwanted side-effects; and the
history of the pill is one of recurrent scares and reassurances
about these side-effects. Most medical anxiety about the pill
is based on the inevitable changes it causes in the chemical
make-up of women taking it. Vast numbers of research
studies throughout the world were summed up in a *Lancet*
leading article which showed that women on the pill have
raised blood levels of iron, copper, cortisone, thyroid hormone, growth hormone and insulin; they have lowered
levels of magnesium, zinc and folic acid; liver function and
the metabolism of sugar and fat are altered; and there are
changes in blood-coagulating factors. All of these changes
can be measured chemically and they are found whether or
not the woman is complaining of any side-effects from the
pill.

Not surprisingly the list of complaints made by women on
the pill is equally long. Probably the most common is gain in
weight, reported by about 10 per cent of women, closely
followed by loss of normal menstruation, reduced sex drive,
depression and headache. Some of these complaints may be
partly psychological in origin – 30 per cent of women given
dummy pills report at least one side-effect – and not every
case of depression in women on the pill is due to the chemical changes it causes; but most of these side-effects are undoubtedly a direct result of the action of the pill on the
body.

What are the long-term hazards of oral contraceptives?
There are probably four really important ones: an increased
risk of thrombosis; a rise in blood pressure that occurs in
some women; chemical diabetes, also found in only some
women; and secondary amenorrhoea.

Thrombosis and the pill

There is no mystery about the pill and thrombosis. One of the two hormones in a combined oral contraceptive is oestrogen, and administration of oestrogen inevitably raises the blood level of at least two of the clotting factors and of fibrinogen, the protein which forms the skeleton of the clot itself. There is an increased risk of spontaneous blood-clotting in any patient given oestrogen – and this has been shown in young women given oestrogen to stop lactation, in older women given oestrogen at the menopause, and in men given the hormone as treatment for cancer of the prostate.

Circumstantial evidence suggesting a link between the pill and thrombosis first began to accumulate in the mid-1960s. By 1970 four large-scale research studies by British doctors had clearly established that a woman who takes an oral contraceptive increases her risk of developing thrombosis by a factor of about four. Further research by staff at the Committee on Safety of Drugs and in Sir Richard Doll's research unit at Oxford University showed that the risk of thrombosis was directly linked with the amount of oestrogen in the pill, and in 1969 the Committee recommended that the amount of oestrogen in pills should be limited to 50 microgrammes. Since then major pharmaceutical companies have further refined their products and many of the newer compounds contain only 30 microgrammes of oestrogen.

Oral contraceptives containing oestrogen are likely to cause thrombosis in any part of the body. Usually the clot forms in the legs, when there is pain and swelling of the calf; less commonly the thrombus spreads up the leg or starts in the lower abdomen, and the dangerous hazard is that a portion of the blood clot may be swept into the heart and lungs. This pulmonary embolism may cause death or progressive shortness of breath. Much less commonly the clot is carried to the brain, where it causes a stroke with resultant paralysis of part of the body. There is less agreement about the effect of the pill on heart disease. Research at Edinburgh

University in the late 1960s and again in 1973 strongly suggested that there was an increased risk of coronary thrombosis among women on the pill; but a larger study in Sweden in 1972 showed no evidence of a link between the two. Both studies agreed that coronary thrombosis in young women is virtually confined to cigarette smokers.

This hazard of blood-clotting is now well recognized and the pill is not prescribed for women with any condition which predisposes them to thrombosis. Most doctors do not regard the presence of varicose veins as a contraindication to the pill.

Continued use of the pill despite the risk of potentially fatal thrombotic side-effects is justified by the very small size of the risk. Of every million women of childbearing age each year four or five die from thromboembolism – fatal complications of venous thrombosis usually starting in the legs. This risk is multiplied by a factor of four to five in women who take the pill; but the twenty to twenty-five deaths each year for every million women is still much less than the risk of death from road accidents (forty-five per million) or breast cancer (200 per million). Furthermore, a woman who switches from the pill to an alternative means of contraception inevitably increases her risk of pregnancy; and as we have seen the risk of death in association with childbearing rises from 200 per million at the age of twenty-five to 600 per million at forty.

High blood pressure

A small proportion of all women who take oral contraceptives develop high blood pressure as a result. The incidence has varied from 2 per cent to 18 per cent in different investigations; but all doctors agree that any woman whose blood pressure rises above normal on the pill should be taken off it and found an alternative contraceptive. This is one of the main justifications for doctors' insistence that the pill should remain on prescription – there are some women whose body chemistry seems very sensitive to changes in its hormonal balance and they can best be identified by regular measurement of the blood pressure.

Raised blood pressure from the pill may not necessarily give rise to any symptoms; indeed, the woman may be unaware of it until her doctor measures the pressure. However, as is emphasized in Chapter 15, any rise in blood pressure above normal is dangerous to health. Fortunately there seems no doubt that when the blood pressure rises as a result of oral contraceptives it usually falls back to normal once the pill is stopped.

Chemical diabetes

The third common medical change in women given oral contraceptives is a tendency towards diabetes. The first sign of the disease diabetes, due to lack of the hormone insulin, is a slowing of the body's response to a carbohydrate meal. In the standard laboratory test a sugary drink is given to a patient and the blood-sugar level measured every thirty minutes for two hours. In a normal individual, sugar is removed from the blood quickly and stored in the liver; in a diabetic the sugar is removed less quickly and the blood level rises to an abnormal level.

This glucose tolerance test is one of the most widely used in medicine and the normal range of results is clearly established. A series of careful studies by Professor Victor Wynn at St Mary's Hospital in London showed that abnormal results were found in up to 80 per cent of women on the pill and the abnormality was marked enough to be described as 'chemical diabetes' in 10–15 per cent of cases. As with raised blood pressure, these changes in sugar metabolism usually caused no symptoms; but there is less agreement about the action that should be advised in these cases. No group of women with chemical diabetes has been kept under observation for long enough to know what if any are the long-term effects; but many doctors believe that any woman with an appreciably abnormal sugar tolerance should be taken off the pill. These metabolic abnormalities are probably much commoner in the small proportion of women whose blood pressure rises in response to oral contraceptives, since both abnormalities indicate unusual sensitivity to the pill.

Amenorrhoea

For the teenager or woman in her twenties probably the most important side-effect of the pill is the one given least publicity – its effect on sexual rhythms. Some time after all the scares about blood-clotting and the pill had died down doctors began to be aware of its possible effects on menstruation, though the first reports of infertility due to the pill had already been made by Professor R. P. Shearman in Australia in 1966. Most women who stop taking the pill resume normal menstruation at once; but in a small proportion periods do not return, and this state of amenorrhoea may persist indefinitely. The absence of periods is due to lack of ovulation, and necessarily means that pregnancy is impossible.

Post-pill amenorrhoea probably affects only one in every 500 women who take oral contraceptives, but it is important in a society when many young women start taking the pill in their teens intending to postpone pregnancy for several years. The condition is almost certainly due to failure of the normal rhythmic release of hormones from the hypothalamus, the part of the brain concerned with sexual activity. Oral contraceptives act partly by blocking the release of these hormones and in some cases the hypothalamus probably does not start to function again when the block is removed. Not surprisingly, there is evidence that post-pill amenorrhoea is more common among women whose periods had been irregular before they started the pill – presumably because of faulty hypothalamic function.

The length of time on the pill seems to be irrelevant, so that there is no scientific basis for the practice of some doctors of taking young women off the pill from time to time 'to re-establish the natural rhythms'. Nor is there any evidence that either the age of the woman or the composition of the pill matter: the condition is a rare, unpredictable hazard. For some doctors the risk of infertility from the pill is sufficiently important for them to advise against its use in women who have had irregular periods and who may wish to become pregnant later on. However, recent research on hypothalamic hormone has made treatment of the condition possible, and it may turn out to be a reversible problem.

Other side-effects

Apart from these four major effects, oral contraceptives increase the liability to a number of disease conditions. These include gall stones, fungus infections of the vagina and cervix, some forms of jaundice and true (biochemical) depression. With most of these disorders the important step for the doctor to take is to recognize the connection with the pill and then to arrange that the woman switches to another contraceptive.

INTRAUTERINE DEVICES

Next to the pill the most reliable form of contraception is an intrauterine device. (Obviously sterilization of one or other partner is 100 per cent reliable, but it is not strictly a form of contraception.) The first attempts to prevent conception by fitting a mechanical device inside the uterus were made before the Second World War, when the German gynaecologist von Gräfenberg introduced the use of a silver ring. Infection was a major problem, however, and it was not until plastics became available that effective intrauterine devices were developed. The early IUDs – the Lippes loop, the Birnberg bow and the Margulies spiral – were tested in North America and Puerto Rico, when it became clear that they were reasonably reliable contraceptive agents but that up to half of women found side-effects such as heavy periods unacceptable.

Technological improvements have led to the introduction of a 'second generation' of IUDs such as the Saf-T-Coil, much smaller than the earlier IUDs, and these are satisfactory in a much higher proportion of cases. The pregnancy rate with these second-generation IUDs has been as low as two per 100 woman-years.

Compared with the pill, IUDs have several advantages: they require no cooperation by the woman; she does not have to remember to take tablets regularly; and there are no secondary changes in the chemical balance of the body. Against this must be set the lower reliability – there is a small but definite risk of pregnancy – and an IUD gives no protection against ectopic pregnancy, in which the fertilized egg starts to grow in the Fallopian tube leading from the ovary to the uterus. Should an unintended pregnancy occur there is an increased risk of miscarriage and other complications. Though there are no side-effects affecting the general health, IUDs can and do cause heavy periods and possibly backache, and there is a slight risk of infection following insertion.

Two long-term anxieties used to be mentioned – the effect on subsequent childbearing and the risk of cancer. What evidence there is suggests that a woman who has never been pregnant does not reduce her chance of proving fertile later if she uses an IUD as a contraceptive for some years; and nothing suggests that even many years' use of an IUD increases the risk of cancer of the uterus later on. However, longer studies are needed before either of these statements can be made with complete certainty.

Some of the newer IUDs such as the Copper 7 and the Gravvigard contain metallic copper, which is known to have a local contraceptive effect. Tests done in research centres in Britain and America have shown that the amount of copper released is very small and that after a month or two of use the device becomes coated with insoluble material and that release of copper then stops. There seems no added risk from the use of copper in these devices.

STERILIZATION

For a couple who have completed their planned family any long-term strategy of birth control should include sterilization of one or other partner. In contrast to medical forms of contraception sterilization almost certainly carries no long-term hazard to health, and has the additional advantages of simplicity, reliability and aesthetic acceptability. As with modern contraceptives, the speed of technological advance has been rapid in the last decade and neither male nor female sterilization is as daunting a procedure as it used to be. Male sterilization, vasectomy, is now carried out under local anaesthetic and takes only fifteen to twenty minutes. The surgeon simply cuts out a section of each of the two vasa (the tubes that carry spermatozoa from the testes to the seminal vesicles, where they are stored until sexual intercourse). In competent hands the operation is very safe: for example, 1,000 vasectomies done at the Family Planning Association's London headquarters in 1972 produced no serious complications and only twenty patients had minor and temporary troubles with the surgeon's incision. It would be wrong to assume, however, that the operation is 100 per cent effective: six of the 1,000 London patients remained fertile and further operation showed that the cut ends of one of the vasa had reunited, and a further section of the tube had to be removed. Another patient who remained fertile was found to have an extra vas on one side. These results show why after a vasectomy surgeons insist on repeated tests before they tell the patient that he can give up the use of contraceptives.

No long-term ill-effects of vasectomy have yet been reported; but it is known that between a quarter and a half of men who have undergone the operation later develop antibodies against their own sperm. This immune reaction probably explains the low success rate of operations designed to reverse vasectomy: even though the plumbing may be restored to normal, the sperm are destroyed by the antibodies.

At present sterilization of women is technically more difficult than it is in men, since the surgeon has to work inside the abdominal cavity. However, a recent invention, the laparoscope, enables him to block the Fallopian tubes by means of an incision only half an inch long, and the operation is now becoming much more widely used. Sterilization of women has now been done for many years, and it is certain that the operation has no adverse effect on the woman's health – indeed the regular hormone cycles and menstrual periods are unaffected.

VENEREAL DISEASE

Venereal disease has been the inescapable partner of sexual promiscuity since time immemorial; and indeed the reason that the great courtesans of history were so rarely pregnant is almost certainly that they quickly acquired gonorrhoea, which made them sterile. Untreated, gonorrhoea may cause no symptoms in a woman but it frequently causes inflammation and later blocking of the Fallopian tubes. Repeated infections in a promiscuous woman virtually always lead to sterility from obstruction to the tubes.

Gonorrhoea is now the most common infectious disease in Europe (other than upper respiratory infections such as the common cold and influenza). There are about 60,000 new cases a year in Britain, but among the sexually most active group, teenagers and adults in their twenties, the rate of infection is about 300 per 100,000. In sexually liberated Scandinavia the rate is nearly 2,000 per 100,000 and in capital cities such as Copenhagen it is several times higher than this.

Symptoms of gonorrhoea in men generally occur within two or three days of exposure to infection; there is pain on passing urine and a discharge from the tip of the penis. Infection may occur without causing any symptoms, however: Dr Joseph Portnoy in Montreal showed in 1974 that as many as 40 per cent of men may be unaware of their infection. Symptomless infection is thought to be more common in women, though anyone who acquires the disease may develop a vaginal discharge and later painful inflammation of the internal genital organs. Gonorrhoea responds quickly and completely to treatment with modern drugs.

The other well-known venereal disease, syphilis, is rare in Britain; there are only 2,000 new cases a year, and half of these occur in male homosexuals. Symptoms of syphilis develop within ten days or so of infection, and the first sign is a hard, painless ulcer at the site of infection. If the disease remains untreated it progresses to a generalized illness – secondary syphilis – which causes headache, sore throat and an extensive rash. Tertiary syphilis affects the heart, brain, spinal cord and nerves (tabes dorsalis; p. 124), and occurs years after the original infection. All forms of syphilis can be treated effectively with penicillin.

Almost as common as gonorrhoea is the new venereal disease, non-specific urethritis. The organisms – whether bacteria or viruses – responsible for this disease have not yet been certainly identified, yet there are about 50,000 cases a year in Britain. Symptoms are similar to those of gonorrhoea, but about 1 per cent of those infected develop arthritis affecting the larger joints together with inflammation of the eyes – a condition called Reiter's syndrome. Unlike other venereal diseases, Reiter's syndrome is not easy to cure, and it may grumble on indefinitely causing permanent damage to joints such as the knees and ankles.

The risk of acquiring venereal disease is clearly related firstly to promiscuity and secondly to the amount of disease in the community. A casual pick-up in a homosexual club in a capital city and a professional prostitute are both likely to be infected; but reports from London venereal disease clinics show the pattern is changing. Ten years ago most men reporting to London clinics had acquired infection from prostitutes; now the most common source is a girlfriend. Another factor thought by many venereologists to be important in explaining the increasing frequency of venereal disease is the change in contraceptive habits. The traditional condom was introduced not as a contraceptive but as a protection against venereal disease – Boswell knew very well that the risks of infection from a prostitute were reduced if he wore 'armour'. As hormone pills and intrauterine devices have become the usual means of contraception among the promiscuous, the protection given by the condom has been lost.

The short answer to the question of risk is that any sexual encounter with a new partner carries a risk of venereal disease. No assurance of health carries any weight, since both men and women can be unaware that they are infected.

SEX AND CANCER

Statistical associations between sexual activity and cancer have been recognized for many years: breast cancer is more common in women who have not had children, for example, and so is cancer of the uterus, whereas cancer of the cervix is more common among women who have had children. When first reported, these associations were thought to be due to changes in hormone production during pregnancy, since female sex hormones such as oestrogen are known to influence the growth of cancers. Recently, however, a much more specific link has been discovered between sex and cancer.

More careful examination of the statistics showed that the risk of cancer of the cervix seems to be more closely linked with sexual activity than with pregnancy. The chance that a woman will develop cervical cancer seems to be increased the earlier she starts sexual activity and the more sexual partners she has. Interrogation of women with this form of cancer confirms that more than might be expected by chance have been sexually promiscuous. Furthermore, while the graph of deaths from cancer of the cervix shows a decline over the last thirty years there is an upswing corresponding to the group of women born between 1911 and 1924. These are the women likely to have been sexually active during the Second World War, when there was a considerable relaxation of sexual taboos. A similar pattern of statistics has been reported for other countries engaged in the war.

Research workers believe that the explanation for this link between sexual promiscuity and cervical cancer is that an infectious agent is involved in its causation, and the most likely culprit is a virus, herpes virus hominis type 2 (HSV 2). This is one of a family of closely related viruses which cause illness in man: the best-known examples are the familiar 'cold sore' on the lips and the painful condition of shingles, but herpes infection of the genital organs is in fact quite common, though it frequently goes unnoticed.

Herpes virus is one of the viruses that seem to be able to cause cancer in animals – it is certainly associated with tumours in frogs, chickens and monkeys. There is some evidence, too, that it is associated with Burkitt's tumour, a cancer of the face and neck that is found in children in central Africa.

Tests in American women with cancer of the cervix show that 98 per cent had evidence of previous infection with herpes virus, compared with only 50 per cent of controls. In such cases the husband may be expected to be a carrier of the virus infection, so it is perhaps not surprising that when husbands of women who have died from cervical cancer remarry, their second wives have a higher-than-normal risk of themselves developing cervical cancer.

Cancer associated with sexual activity is not solely a female problem. Though there is less conclusive evidence, there is some suggestion that cancer of the prostate in men is also linked with promiscuity and occurs more often among men who started sexual activity at an early age and who have had many sex partners. Again the likely explanation is that the cancer is linked with infection with HSV 2.

THE BALANCE

The only form of sexual activity which comes out as un-equivocally hazardous in terms of health is promiscuity. A man or woman who has a large number of sexual partners is at risk of acquiring venereal disease and may be more likely to develop prostatic cancer if a man and cervical cancer if a woman. On the other hand, Hilaire Belloc observed that the only persons who seemed content on their death-beds were those who had spent their lives in the 'unremitting pursuit of sexual pleasure'.

Chapter 14

PROSPECTS FOR ONE'S CHILDREN

ONE of the most important factors determining the prospects of the individual child occurs at conception, when the genes in the mother's and father's sex cells are united into one cell. Since they develop from this single cell every other cell in the body contains duplicate pairs of genes – some 50,000 – and these are responsible for characteristics such as eye colour, intelligence or height. Occasionally the absence of or abnormality of a gene may cause disease, such as haemophilia (an inadequate clotting mechanism in the blood) and sickle-cell anaemia (occurring mainly in Negroes, whose red blood cells may contain an abnormal type of haemoglobin). But usually the hereditary tendency to develop a particular illness or abnormality is governed by several genes, and environmental factors also play a considerable part. For example, in coronary heart disease (p. 298) several environmental factors – cigarette smoking, exercise and diet among others – act over long periods on a genetically susceptible individual.

This chapter does not cover heredity (which needs a book to itself) but deals with the possible effects of the mother's environment, health and treatment and the course of her pregnancy on her baby, both before and shortly after birth. But first we consider two sorts of hazard a baby can face: premature birth and congenital abnormalities.

PREMATURE BABIES

In the United Kingdom about 7 per cent of all newborn babies are 'premature', weighing under 2,500 grammes. About two thirds of these are truly premature or 'pre-term' –

that is, they are born before thirty-seven completed weeks from the first day of the mother's last menstrual period. The cause of early birth is usually unknown (though it may be due to multiple pregnancy or bleeding in the womb). The 'pre-term' baby faces difficulties in breathing, feeding and maintaining body temperature and runs an increased risk of suffering from jaundice and bleeding into the brain. These complications are more likely the earlier the child is born.

The other third of premature babies are 'small-for-dates', having birth weights abnormally low for the length of pregnancy. Growth may have been restricted because of foetal malformations, infections during pregnancy (including rubella), severe maternal malnutrition, toxaemia of pregnancy and multiple pregnancy. The smaller babies born to mothers who smoke during pregnancy (p. 246) also fall into this category. In this group of babies the main risks are of oxygen shortage (both before and during birth) and the effects of a low blood-sugar level after birth – which presumably results from the baby's malnutrition during pregnancy.

The baby's birth weight is an important milestone in its development. In the first month of life the death rate is twenty-five times as high in babies weighing under 2,500 grammes at birth as in normal-weight babies; their incidence of serious disease of the nervous system – cerebral palsy, severe mental retardation, blindness and epilepsy – is three times that of normal babies, and is particularly high in those weighing under 1,500 grammes. Both groups of premature babies are affected, but pre-term babies are especially likely to become spastics and small-for-date babies to develop epilepsy or mental retardation. In later childhood premature babies tend to be lighter, less intelligent, more often admitted to hospital for illness, and have a higher incidence of visual, hearing and other defects. This difference is shown particularly vividly in the case of twins with a birth-weight difference of 300 grammes or more: the undersized twin continues to be inferior in both physical growth and intelligence (with an IQ difference of about 5) even into adult life.

Recent research, however, has shown that careful attention to diet and temperature may enable many even very low birth-weight babies to survive without obvious brain damage. Frequent, small milk feeds given by stomach tube will prevent the blood-sugar level falling to a dangerously low figure. If the baby is also kept in a warm incubator, most of this food can be made available for growth – particularly of the brain – instead of having to be used to produce heat for the body. Finally, rearing plays a very important part in the way even an apparently normal premature baby grows up: one study of five-year-olds showed that though children brought up in a normal home had little handicap, those exposed to communal family stresses were five times as likely to be unsettled or maladjusted as non-premature children. (See also p. 17.)

CONGENITAL ABNORMALITIES

At birth almost everybody has some sort of minor abnormality, or anomaly, such as a hairy mole on the skin or webbing of one of the fingers or toes. About 2 per cent of babies, however, have a major congenital abnormality, such as cleft palate or spina bifida. Moreover, most experts now believe that this figure underestimates the true incidence of severe deformities in pregnancy; in the early stages this may be ten times that seen in stillborn or liveborn infants, but the pregnancy is terminated early on by spontaneous miscarriage.

We know some of the general influences leading to foetal malformations, such as geography and social class, but we are still ignorant of the specific causes. Compression of the baby inside the womb may cause a few deformities – including club foot, dislocation of the hip and cleft palate – while internal bands may constrict the baby's limbs. Recently more attention has been given to outside events during pregnancy. At one time stories that particular abnormalities were linked to external factors, including various medicines or foods, were dismissed as old wives' tales. But the discovery in 1939 that rubella (German measles) in the mother early in pregnancy could cause gross abnormalities in the baby opened up a whole new field of research into these factors, or 'teratogens'. Added impetus was given by the finding that not only could X-ray examination of the pregnant woman increase the risk of abnormalities, and of leukaemia in the baby, but that an apparently harmless sleeping tablet, thalidomide, had caused an 'epidemic' of a particularly rare and striking deformity. In 1960–61 thalidomide probably caused an eighty-fold incidence in phocomelia (absence or shortening of one or more of the limbs) in countries where it was used – in some without a doctor's prescription. Though apparently only a fifth of mothers who took thalidomide gave birth to deformed children, probably as many as 10,000 children were affected by it, and half of them survived. This led to attempts to link medicines given to the pregnant mother with congenital abnormalities in her baby, and also studies of the effect of any procedure or treatment during pregnancy.

We now recognize that various factors may produce different effects at different stages of pregnancy: in the first three months they will tend to produce structural abnormalities, while in the last three months they will tend to affect foetal functions. These factors may act directly on the foetus, the placenta or uterus (womb), or indirectly by affecting the hormone balance in the mother. At least one agent (the sex hormone, oestrogen) is now known to have very delayed effects on the offspring which are not revealed until adolescence. Finally, there is a suggestion that taking the contraceptive pill before pregnancy may upset the mother's metabolism in some cases and make her baby more likely to develop jaundice when being breast-fed.

We now also recognize three main principles in how these factors work in pregnancy. Firstly, small amounts of various substances may produce gross damage in the foetus but apparently do the mother no harm. Secondly, the foetal re-

sponse may be closely related to the dose of the drug: very
small doses may have no effect, larger ones produce malformations, and still larger ones kill the embryo. Thirdly, the
stage of pregnancy at which these factors operate may be the
important feature: given at the same stage in pregnancy, a
wide variety of influences (infections, X-rays and drugs) will
produce the same deformity.

GENERAL ENVIRONMENT

From the work of Professor Thomas McKeown and his research team at Birmingham we know that there are wide
differences between various countries in the incidence of
various deformities and, even more interestingly, that there
are also differences between various parts of the same country; between different years; between different times of the
year; and between different social classes. Defects of the brain
and spinal cord – particularly absence of the brain (anencephaly) and spina bifida – are eight times more common in
South Wales than in Japan. In England and Wales the death
rate from these deformities in babies up to a year old is much
higher in the north and west than in the south and east –
while in the mining valleys of South Wales the figure is
double that in the coastal plain. These geographical variations cannot be explained by differences in social class
structure alone. In Dublin the peak rate for anencephaly, in
1960–61, was three times the trough rate, in 1944–5, and
similar swings with time have been found in the USA, Scotland and Birmingham. Some areas also show a seasonal variation – the incidence of stillbirths from anencephaly being
highest in December and lowest in May.

Other research has shown that anencephaly is three times
as common in unskilled workers (social class V) as in the
professional classes (social class I). Spina bifida and anencephaly are also commoner in first and fourth and subsequent births than in second and third births – though the

show little link with the mother's age. Maternal age is, in fact, only conclusively relevant in one birth abnormality: mongolism, or Down's syndrome, in which it is roughly ten times as common in babies born to mothers aged forty and over as in those of twenty-nine and under. An unexplained finding is that the incidence of two conditions, haemophilia and achondroplasia (a type of dwarfism), rises with increasing *paternal* age.

The considerable variations in the frequency of defects of this kind from year to year have led authorities such as Sir Dugald Baird to suggest that nutritional factors may also be relevant, and that the critical period is the pregnancy that led to the birth of the mother and her early years. Sir Dugald, a distinguished Aberdeen obstetrician, has shown that the incidence of these abnormal births has varied considerably this century, and that it reached its peak in Britain in the late 1950s and early 1960s, when the women having babies were those born during the depression in the 1930s. The hypothesis is supported by his finding that the abnormality rate began its rise for women aged fifteen to nineteen in 1946, for those aged twenty to twenty-four in 1951, and for those aged twenty-five to twenty-nine in 1956. Such a theory would fit in with the known association of spina bifida with socio-economic circumstances.

POOR MATERNAL HEALTH AND DIET

Women whose health is less than perfect – what the World Health Organization calls 'positive health' – tend to have small babies. Doctors set the level of low birth weight in a baby as under 2,500 grammes, and birth weight below that level is the direct cause of, or is associated with, 80–90 per cent of infant deaths, while up to a third of the survivors have mental handicap and other abnormalities. The mother most likely to have a low-birth-weight ('premature') baby is a young girl in her first pregnancy who has had little or no medical care during pregnancy and who comes from an underprivileged group, works hard and eats badly. This generalization emphasizes that the causes are multiple, if often linked; other associations with prematurity include a maternal age of over forty and short stature. Stature is related to social class: about half the women from the two upper classes are 5 ft 4 in. or more tall, compared with only a fifth of those in the lowest social class, and the mother's social status has a paramount role in prematurity. Low status is associated with early and rapidly repeated childbearing, which is continued until the mother is relatively old. In mothers of low status the risk of prematurity rises after the second birth, while in middle-class mothers it remains low for all births after the first. In this way begins the 'cycle of deprivation' – low social status; early childbearing; impoverished childhood in all its senses; continuation of low social status – which many have emphasized as one of the major evils in our present-day society.

Even so, this view of the formation of a lower social caste from which there is no escape has been challenged because it ignores another important factor in inheritance – that is, 'regression to the mean'. By this is meant the tendency of children to be more average than their parents – for example, with intelligence (on which most of the studies have been done) the children of very bright parents are less bright than they, though still brighter than average; whereas the children of very dull parents are less dull than they, but still duller than average. In the population this reshuffling of genes leaves the distribution of the intelligence quotient constant, but in individual families it entails a continual rise and fall in intelligence of succeeding generations. In their turn, these changes underlie movement from one social class to another, which in Britain Professor H. J. Eysenck has estimated amounts to about 30 per cent: bright children rise and dull ones fall in the social scale. Regression also plays an important part in the inheritance of other features which are strongly controlled by genetic causes, such as height.

The mother's diet during pregnancy may also have an important effect on her baby. In malnourished communities such as those in developing countries both miscarriages and stillbirths are commoner than in developing ones. Many stillbirths are due to premature birth, and a poor maternal diet particularly after the sixth month of pregnancy is known to make this more likely. Compared with babies born to normally nourished mothers, those born to malnourished ones (especially when the diet contains little first-class protein) have a greater tendency to be anaemic and to have less well developed bones and teeth. There are also more pregnancy complications in malnourished mothers. In particular, toxaemia – high blood pressure, ankle-swelling and urinary abnormalities – is commoner, and this in turn may affect the foetus.

There has been much argument about the effect of a poor maternal diet on the brain of the unborn child. The brain grows most rapidly from the seventh month of foetal life to the second year of age, and, though it is less affected by malnutrition than body growth, a severely deprived maternal diet may cause the baby to be born with a smaller brain than normal and probably with learning handicaps. Given a normal diet after birth – particularly if combined with maternal and social stimulation – many malnourished children may show a remarkable catch-up in mental development. Nevertheless, effects of this kind are related to very poor diets and are unlikely to affect foetal development in most communities in the developed countries.

ILLNESSES IN THE MOTHER

The most notorious maternal illness is rubella: between the vital third and eighth weeks of foetal development this may produce serious deformities, including cataract, deafness and mental retardation. But other infections during pregnancy may have equally serious consequences: for example, live mumps virus, given as a vaccine, will produce similar effects.

The virus known as cytomegalovirus, or CMV, may produce little or no upset in the mother but a serious illness in the baby, including jaundice, a small-sized head and mental deficiency: some 5–15 per cent of all cases of mental retardation are said to be due to this cause. A similarly serious disease of the brain and eyes may be produced by toxoplasmosis – infection within the womb by the protozoal parasite *Toxoplasma gondii,* which in the mother may cause only a trivial upset or an illness similar to glandular fever.

Infections which are usually more obvious in the mother and which produce illness in the baby include syphilis (causing a wide range of abnormalities), gonorrhoea (which may cause blindness in the newborn baby through infection acquired in the birth canal) and smallpox.

Other types of maternal illness in later pregnancy may also have important effects on the foetus. Women with established diabetes or a tendency to develop the disease tend to have large babies. The incidence of malformations in these babies also seems slightly higher than normal, but the chief risk is of sudden death in the foetus relatively late in pregnancy, possibly due to inadequate functioning of the placenta. For this reason the modern management of diabetic pregnancy now often includes scrupulous control of diabetes, careful timing of delivery (usually being started artificially two or three weeks early), and intensive care of the baby during and after labour – all of which has greatly decreased the death rate in these babies. Other important maternal factors affecting the placenta are high blood pressure, prolonged pregnancy and bleeding into the uterus. Again, this may kill the baby or may deprive it of sufficient oxygen and cause permanent brain damage. Various difficulties and complications during labour itself may have a similar effect. Moreover, the effects of any of these factors are greatly increased in premature infants.

DRUGS TAKEN DURING PREGNANCY

It is important to emphasize that only one in every twenty birth abnormalities appears to be due to a known teratogen. Some of the latter are infections, but since the thalidomide tragedy there has been much publicity about drugs taken during pregnancy. Much of our knowledge about the role of these has come from a large-scale study by Professor John Forfar and his colleagues in the Edinburgh University Department of Child Health. Their research findings highlight just how commonly mothers take medicines during pregnancy: of 1,369 mothers, 97 per cent had taken drugs prescribed by the doctor and 65 per cent ones bought over the counter. Compared with the mothers of normal babies, more of those who had had children with congenital deformities had taken aspirin, stomach powders, appetite suppressants, barbiturates, cough medicines, iron, sulphonamides and vitamins. Other research has also convincingly indicted antileukaemia, antiepilepsy and antithyroid drugs; sex hormones; the antibiotic tetracycline (which stains the teeth and reversibly impairs bone growth in the unborn baby); iodides (which may be found in some cough mixtures bought over the counter); and quinine. But most mothers in Professor Forfar's study produced healthy babies, and we still do not know how much weight to put on these apparent links. The value of his survey is to make doctors and pregnant mothers alike ask whether any drug is really necessary.

All teratogens produce major damage in the embryo between the third and the eighth week of development – often before the woman realizes that she is pregnant. Thus between days thirty-four and thirty-nine of development major deformities are likely in the ears and head; between days thirty-nine and forty-three in the arms; between days forty-three and forty-six in the legs; and after day forty-six minor abnormalities may occur in the thumbs. The type of effect produced depends not only on the time at which the drug is given, but also for how long: large doses of vitamin D given to pregnant women cause a particular type of abnormality in a heart valve, smaller ones merely poor enamel on the teeth. Even so, since most of the mothers taking drugs studied by Professor Forfar produced normal children, any effect they have is small.

But we are still scratching the surface of the problem, as shown by the discovery only in 1971 that a hormone taken by mothers during pregnancy might be associated with an unusual type of cancer developing in their daughters at adolescence or even later. Doctors in the USA identified fourteen girls aged between fifteen and twenty-two years with cancer of the vagina: all except one of the mothers had taken large doses of stilboestrol early in pregnancy to try to prevent miscarriage. This treatment had been given in 1945–51 and is no longer used (it was never popular in Britain), so fortunately it seems unlikely that further cases will occur. Nevertheless, the incident reveals that cancer-producing substances may cross the placenta and cause disease many years later, and that only a small proportion of the children at risk are affected. For this reason keeping careful records of human malformations can play a vital part in identifying such links. New drugs are, of course, now tested in pregnant animals, but these may not react in the same way as man and such tests would not detect any long-term effects such as that of stilboestrol.

The tissues of the foetus deal with drugs less well than those of the mother, a factor which becomes particularly important just before birth and during labour. For example, long-acting sulpha drugs taken by the mother for a urinary infection may cross the placenta and cause serious jaundice in the baby; similarly, tetracyclines stain the teeth and slow down the growth of the bones, though the latter is reversible. Some anaesthetics given to the mother during labour may depress breathing in the baby or reduce the blood flow in its body. Similar, though longer-lasting, effects may be seen in babies born to mothers addicted to morphine, heroin and barbiturate sleeping pills: the babies may be restless, cry excessively, have disturbed sleep, and need treatment for four to eight weeks if they are not to develop convulsions and die.

OTHER MATERNAL INFLUENCES

Chronic alcoholism may be associated with retardation of growth and deformities of the face, eyes and heart and blood-vessels; there is no evidence, however, that a single alcoholic binge can have this effect, even though according to tradition bridal couples in Carthage were exhorted not to drink alcohol on their wedding day.

A few years ago it was also suggested that maternal influenza might double the risk of leukacmia developing in the child after birth, but there is now known to be no statistical foundation for this. But one factor, X-irradiation, does increase the risk of leukaemia: babies born to mothers who were exposed to the blast of the atomic bombs at Hiroshima or Nagasaki developed leukaemia about eight times as commonly as normally, while an Oxford survey showed that babies born to mothers who had had diagnostic X-ray films taken during pregnancy had double the risk (p. 209).

Incompatibility between the tissues of mother and foetus may cause haemolytic disease of the newborn, with serious anaemia, jaundice and brain damage. This occurs when the baby's blood group is different from that of the mother – usually the mother is rhesus group negative and the baby rhesus positive; the mother produces antibodies against the rhesus factor which cross the placenta into the baby's bloodstream and damage its red blood cells. Occasionally the incompatibility affects the blood group A system, but here its effects are usually milder. Not only can rhesus haemolytic disease of the newborn now be treated effectively, but more recently doctors have been able to start a prevention programme, giving injections to stop rhesus antibodies forming in the mother.

A recent and widely publicized possible link early in pregnancy was between eating blighted potatoes and spina bifida. Subsequent research has not confirmed this suggestion, but another survey is now going on into a possible association between birth deformities and maternal exposure to anaesthetic gases in surgical operating theatres – as occurs, for instance, in anaesthetists or nurses.

Despite all this research, however, Professor McKeown has concluded that, though things are likely to get better through early diagnosis of severe malformations (offering the mother therapeutic abortion) and better treatment of babies born with them, we are unlikely ever to have much control over these environmental influences.

In that fine and private place, the womb, the environmental influences at work are likely to remain obscure and unpredictable accidents occurring at the time of fertilization or implantation during early foetal development due in part, perhaps, to minor disturbances of delicately balanced maternal metabolic factors beyond our control.

Moreover, it is important to realize how difficult it is in most cases to make a firm correlation between events during pregnancy and birth deformities: careful and large-scale surveys have to be done before suggestions can be proved or disproved. On the one hand, it is obviously important to explore the role of any possible teratogen, even though these probably account for less than 5 per cent of all developmental abnormalities. On the other, the need not to alarm mothers unnecessarily about effects in pregnancy can hardly be over-emphasized.

Chapter 15

THE VITAL STATISTICS
OF DEATH

DESPITE the flood of TV programmes, magazine features and newspaper articles on medical topics, there are still widespread misconceptions about the most serious risks to life – even among the readers of 'quality' newspapers and books. Cancer, for example, is mistakenly believed to be the most important cause of death in adult life, yet heart disease and stroke each account for more deaths. There are hard facts about the major causes of death, and some of them have been discussed in earlier chapters. But as a postscript it seems worthwhile reviewing the major killing conditions at each stage of life and sorting out fact from fiction. Inevitably this will repeat and expand some of the facts given in other chapters in the book, but in a different context.

BIRTH DEFECTS

By far the most important causes of death in the first four years of life are congenital anomalies and birth injuries (lumped together by the Registrar General for practical reasons). One child in every fifty has a major birth defect (p. 278). One of the most ancient traditions of folklore – older than any formal system of medicine – is the belief that birth abnormalities may be linked with a mother's experiences in pregnancy (p. 278). In common with all diseases, congenital abnormalities are the result of the interplay between the genetic make-up of the individual and external circumstances. Better understanding of the mechanisms of inheritance in recent years has made it possible for genetic counsellors to give advice to parents who are apprehensive because there is a family history of some birth abnormality or because they themselves have had an abnormal child. More accurate forecasting can sometimes be combined with antenatal diagnosis, so that with parents who run an increased risk of having a child with, say, Down's syndrome (mongolism) – a common form of mental retardation known to be associated with an abnormality of the chromosomes – a test can be done early in pregnancy. If this shows that the foetus is indeed abnormal the mother can be offered the choice of termination of the pregnancy. Similarly, if the condition is known to be sex-linked – such as some forms of muscular dystrophy – the mother can be offered the chance of termination of pregnancy if the foetus is male (and likely to be affected) but not if it is female and so cannot be affected.

Despite all the research effort expended on the subject, we are still almost entirely in the dark about the environmental factors that cause congenital malformations (including mental and biochemical as well as physical abnormalities). The thalidomide tragedy stressed the role of drugs and other chemicals as a cause of foetal abnormalities: yet no more than 2–3 per cent of all the congenital defects are due to drugs such as aminopterin and cortisone or to chemical agents such as mercury or polyvinyl chloride. Nationally and internationally, streamlined, computer-based monitoring systems were set up after the thalidomide tragedy to give early warning of drugs or environmental agents with an adverse effect on the foetus, but so far they have all failed to come up with even one substance not previously known to have a teratogenic action. In part, of course, this failure is good news – perhaps there are no other teratogens as potent as thalidomide; and in part it reflects the difficulty of detecting small changes in rare events. To incriminate a substance that doubles the frequency of a birth defect that normally occurs at a rate of once in every 1,000 births (a very high rate indeed) it would be necessary to study 23,000 births.

There has been one real advance in the last decade, and that is the reduction in the toll of birth abnormalities due to infection of the expectant mother with rubella (German measles). Vaccination of teenage girls as a routine has combined with readier availability of therapeutic abortion to reduce the numbers of children with heart disease or deafness due to intrauterine rubella.

Rubella is not the only infection that can damage the foetus, however: cytomegalovirus and toxoplasmosis – two other mild illnesses as they affect children and adults – can cause blindness or mental retardation in the foetus if infection occurs during pregnancy. One recent estimate suggested that between 200 and 600 babies born each year in Britain have mental retardation due to cytomegalovirus infection before birth. Fortunately there are good prospects that a vaccine will soon be available for this condition, too. Again, however, these infections account for only a small proportion of all congenital anomalies – probably less than 2 per cent – so that between them drugs, known environmental poisons such as mercury, and infections can be implicated in less than 5 per cent of congenital defects.

While no single cause can be pinpointed for the great mass of congenital abnormalities, there is a lot of evidence on factors known to be relevant. For instance, there are very wide geographical variations in the incidence of defects such as spina bifida (see chapter 4). Spina bifida – failure of normal development of the spine and spinal cord – is one of the most common serious birth defects and has been studied in great detail in countries throughout the world. The geographical variations in its incidence seem to be linked with the softness of water supplies (p. 53), but as yet no explanation can be offered for this effect.

After congenital deformities, the most common causes of death in infancy are the infections – pneumonia, gastroenteritis and virus infections. These reflect the vulnerability of the small child to infection, and indeed it is this category of deaths in infancy that has been so nearly eliminated in the twentieth century and so produced the population explosion. Better sanitation and the ready availability of dried milk have helped to conquer gastroenteritis; while measles, diphtheria and the other killing fevers have been controlled by immunization. Three other conditions warrant mention – 'cot death', battered babies and leukaemia.

SUDDEN DEATH IN INFANCY

Each year in Britain nearly 2,000 infants under a year old die suddenly and unexpectedly, usually in their cots at night – hence the familiar phrase 'cot death'. Cot death is now, indeed, the most common cause of death between the age of one month and one year. Though by definition these deaths are unexpected, in many cases they are not unexplained. Recent refinements in forensic techniques have made it possible to incriminate a virus illness in about one third of such deaths, while others can be shown to be due to inhalation of vomit or an unsuspected defect in the heart; but a solid block of the deaths, perhaps a third or more, remain a mystery. As so often where medical science is baffled, a rag-bag of statistical associations has been collected over the years, some of which may be pointers to an explanation. Cot deaths occur more often among under-privileged children – those living in circumstances of overcrowding, with poor nutrition, poor obstetric record, small birth weights and a tendency for mothers not to seek medical advice or to attend child welfare clinics. There is a seasonal incidence, with a peak in the winter and a low-point in August. As with heart disease and birth defects, there is an association between infant mortality and soft water. There is some evidence of a link between cot deaths and magnesium deficiency in the diet. Another possible dietary factor is vitamin E deficiency. A recent theory, advanced in October 1974, is that some of the deaths are due to chemical disturbances caused by feeding infants with too concentrated dried milk mixtures.

More generally, some minor illness such as a snuffly cold has been noted in nearly half of the cases in the two weeks preceding death. Again, in nearly half of the deaths the child has been in hospital, or has been under medical care in the week before death. However, there is no question of serious illness being missed by ineffectual parents: most infants seem to have been healthy or only mildly unwell on the day before death. 'Death occurs silently, suddenly and unobserved, usually during sleep, the child being found lifeless, without evidence of struggle, on average six hours after last being seen alive.' That comment by the *British Medical Journal* in 1974 sums up the lack of hard knowledge on the subject.

Battering of small babies to death by the parents or guardians has been recognized as a major problem only within the last fifteen years. How many infants die from this cause each year is still a matter of dispute: it is certainly several hundred. Only too often, however, the evidence is no more than suggestive: in a recent series of deaths investigated in Birmingham open verdicts were recorded in nearly half, though the medical and social teams had no doubt about the circumstances (p. 18).

Most of the factors associated with sudden, unexplained death in infancy seem to act as risk factors for battering, too: but in addition there is clear evidence that the problem is more frequent when the parents are young, socially isolated, of low intelligence and with 'personality disorders'. At present all that can be done is to attempt to recognize the condition on the first occasion that the baby is assaulted and then for the medical and social workers to act resolutely and effectively to prevent further episodes.

LEUKAEMIA IN CHILDHOOD

Childhood leukaemia is one of the most feared of all diseases, largely because until quite recently the diagnosis was a sentence of death. This is no longer the case. With expert treatment and early diagnosis a child found to have the common type of leukaemia in 1976 has at least a one in four chance of permanent cure, and this chance is being improved year by year. The very real progress that has been made in treatment has not been matched, however, by equal advances in understanding of the cause of the condition. Leukaemia may be transmitted by virus infection in animals, and in cats and mice this seems to be the common means of transmission of the disease; but there is no evidence that virus infection plays a major part in the cause of human leukaemia. In particular there is no convincing evidence to link childhood leukaemia with household pets – despite reports in the late 1960s that cat leukaemia might be infectious for man.

Several careful studies have been done in attempts to detect 'clustering' in leukaemia; but again the tendency for cases of leukaemia to occur more often among contacts of children with the disease has been very slight or non-existent. If there is an infectious agent that has a part in the causation of human leukaemia it seems likely to play a very minor part.

At present, indeed, only one factor has been proved of importance in the causation of leukaemia – radiation. Quite early in this century it became clear that doctors and scientists working with X-rays greatly increased their chances of developing leukaemia, and more recently the risk has been measured with greater accuracy. In the later 1950s Alice Stewart and her colleagues at Oxford showed that children whose mothers had been X-rayed during pregnancy for any reason had nearly double the normal risk of developing leukaemia (or some other childhood cancer) during the first ten years of life. This risk seems to be higher in children who catch infections such as whooping cough or measles during the first four years of life. This is probably not because of any link between leukaemia and the virus causing the illness, but simply that children born with less than average natural resistance to infections have a similar diminished resistance to leukaemia. Such a hypothesis is supported by the finding that children under four with asthma and a history of X-ray exposure before birth have about twenty-five times the 'normal' risk of leukaemia. Current medical policy is, of course, to avoid all X-ray exposure during pregnancy unless it is absolutely essential.

Japanese who were children in Hiroshima and Nagasaki when the atomic bombs were dropped in 1945 have an increased risk of leukaemia. Of 15,000 children aged less than ten who survived the bombing, sixteen died of leukaemia or other cancers in the succeeding twenty-five years, as opposed to an expected figure of less than two. As yet, of course, these children are still well below the age at which cancer is common, so the full effects of their irradiation may not yet have become apparent.

These effects of the Japanese bombs raise the question of the effects of atomic tests on health. The subject has been argued endlessly, but the current expert opinion is unanimous that any increase in the amount of radioactive material in the atmosphere increases the number of cases of leukaemia that occur each year. Perhaps a single 'clean' test may be responsible for only a handful of cases worldwide; but some extra deaths are an inevitable result of every atmospheric test.

SCHOOLCHILDREN AND TEENAGERS

Once children have passed the age of five most of those going to die in infancy from disorders present at birth will have done so, and medically they should be in the safest period of their lives. Sadly, between the ages of five and twenty-four the most common cause of death is injury in road accidents – and here Britain's record is poor compared with many other developed countries.

In proportion to the population at risk Britain has the worst record in Western Europe for deaths among child pedestrians. To be strictly accurate, the statistics show that Britain has the worst figures for children up to the age of five and from ten to fourteen, but Western Germany has a slightly worse record for the six- to nine-year-olds. Britain has proportionally four times the numbers of child pedestrian casualties under the age of six as does France. This black record is almost entirely due to injuries in built-up areas, where 73 per cent of casualties occur; and the risk is especially high in older cities where traffic density is high and socio-economic conditions are poor. Commenting on these figures in 1973, the *British Medical Journal* observed that it may be significant that 'the United Kingdom is the only technically developed country in Europe where pedestrians are allowed to cross the road whenever, wherever and however they like'.

EARLY ADULT LIFE

Road accidents now account for almost half of all deaths of men between the ages of fifteen and twenty-four in the technically developed countries of Europe. In addition to the deaths, many thousands of young men and women are permanently crippled every year. In contrast to the children, most of these teenagers and young adults are either drivers or passengers of cars or motorcycles – in this age range more private car users are killed than pedestrians. In the decade 1961–70 the increase in pedestrian deaths was 10 per cent but the figure for private car users was 86 per cent.

Some halt in the rising numbers of killed and injured motorists came from the Road Safety Act 1967, which introduced blood and breath tests for the detection of excess alcohol in drivers – some years after similar legislation had been introduced in other countries. The year after the Act came into force road deaths dropped by 15 per cent – a saving of over 1,000 lives. In the dangerous period between 10 p.m. and 4 a.m. casualties were reduced by 33 per cent. Since 1968 deaths and injuries have begun to rise again, but there is good evidence that the drinking-and-driving legislation is still having a beneficial effect, and it seems likely that very soon these regulations will be made still more effective.

The legal requirement that seat-belts should be fitted to all vehicles has also had a useful effect in reducing the severity of injuries in car users, but again Britain has lagged behind other countries in making their use compulsory. No one doubts the value of seat-belts; and when, for example, the Australian State of Victoria made their use compulsory in 1971, the following twelve months saw a drop in road deaths of 12·5 per cent compared with annual rises of 5 per cent in the previous years.

One type of accident in which seat-belts give little protection is the high-speed collision between a private car and a lorry. These collisions account for many of the deaths in accidents on motorways and link roads – in one study at Birmingham Accident Hospital 40 per cent of 564 deaths of vehicle occupants came from car–lorry collisions, though cars outnumber lorries by seven to one. Experts estimate that in such accidents there is 95 per cent risk of injury to the car occupants and virtually none to the lorry-driver or his passengers. Whereas seat-belts prevent 50 per cent of injuries in car accidents the figure falls to 20 per cent for car–lorry collisions and less than 10 per cent when cars run into the rear of lorries. Professor William Gissane, director of the Road Injuries Research Group at the Birmingham Accident Hospital, argues that cars and lorries should be segregated on to separate roads – or perhaps heavy transport should be transferred to rail rather than road.

Between the ages of twenty-one and forty, motor accidents remain the principal cause of death, but second place is held by suicide. It is important to distinguish suicide from attempted suicide, sometimes called 'parasuicide' by psychiatrists. Suicide is in fact common as a cause of death among elderly men, who tend to hang, drown or gas themselves; whereas in contrast suicidal attempts are most prevalent in young girls who take an overdose of sleeping-pills or tranquillizers. Nevertheless, while ten times as many men in the age group sixty-five to sixty-nine kill themselves each year as do young men aged twenty to twenty-five, suicide ranks as a major killer only in younger men, since deaths from natural causes are so much rarer before the age of forty. Furthermore some at least of the older suicides kill themselves because they know they are dying from a fatal disease.

In the last ten years there has been a dramatic rise in the frequency of admissions to hospital for attempted suicide, which is now in many hospitals the most common cause of emergency medical admission, probably accounting for about 100,000 such admissions in hospitals in Britain, with the numbers continuing to rise (p. 31).

MIDDLE AGE

After the age of forty two conditions dominate the mortality statistics: coronary thrombosis and stroke. It is an extraordinary fact that coronary thrombosis, by far the most important cause of death in middle age in all technically advanced countries, did not even appear in many medical textbooks in the 1920s. In part this was due to failure by doctors to recognize that the condition existed – though perfectly accurate descriptions of the characteristic pain of angina pectoris had been written by physicians in the eighteenth and nineteenth centuries – but the unfamiliarity of the condition also reflected its rarity. Coronary thrombosis, a rare and esoteric disorder in 1924, is now so common that one man in five develops its symptoms by the age of sixty-five in Britain and by sixty in the USA. Over 100,000 men and women die from coronary thrombosis each year in Britain; and between the ages of forty-one and sixty deaths from this one condition outnumber those from the total of stroke, bronchitis, and lung, stomach and breast cancers. Such a preponderance cannot be explained simply by the medical conquest of infectious diseases such as tuberculosis and pneumonia. Coronary thrombosis has become common in the last fifty years because of some change in our way of life in advanced, Western countries. Yet despite vast amounts of research in Europe and the USA there is no general agreement about the explanation: there are supporters for dietary theories, behaviourist theories and environmental poisoning theories, and those who combine all three together.

Diet undoubtedly is one of the factors – see Chapter 2 (p. 44). A high-calorie diet containing large amounts of animal fat will certainly increase the incidence of coronary thrombosis in a population. How much importance should be given to sugar, to fat and to cholesterol is still disputed among the experts. Some experts argue that the lack of natural fibre in the processed, refined Western diet is an important factor; one Norwegian professor, Victor Linden, has recently suggested that the culprit is vitamin D added to foods such as margarine and swallowed as vitamin pills. Diet alone, however, is unlikely to be the major factor except in cases where overeating leads to grossly excessive weight and in the small minority of persons born with a tendency to high fat levels in the blood – familial hypercholesterolaemia.

The behaviourists argue that the unique feature of modern society is its combination of emotional stress with physical inactivity. Anger, fear, irritation and excitement all have similar effects on the body: it prepares itself for vigorous muscular action by speeding up the heart and releasing fats and sugars into the bloodstream for use as instant energy. If nevertheless the body remains seated in a chair or a car seat the system has to wind down unused, and the fats are deposited on the walls of the blood-vessels, narrowing their calibre and increasing the likelihood of thrombosis. This chain of physical events explains the high incidence of coronary thrombosis among Type A individuals – ambitious, aggressive, impatient, go-ahead persons so typical of the stereotype of the executive cut down in his prime by a heart attack. Again, however, the explanation cannot account for all the increase in coronary deaths, which also occur among relaxed, non-ambitious drop-outs from the rat race.

Behaviourist explanations also include the theory that the physical inactivity of modern civilized life holds the key. While our ancestors (or at least the wealthy section of society in early centuries) may have gorged themselves on meat, eggs, butter, cheese and alcohol, they also rode on horseback, walked, fenced and generally maintained a high level of physical activity. In contrast, the furthest some businessmen walk is down the stairs to their cars, unless they play golf – and even then they may use an electric golf-buggy. Recent work at the London School of Hygiene (p. 103) has shown that men who take regular, vigorous physical exercise cut their risk of coronary thrombosis to about one third of that in men of the same age, smoking habits and build who do no more than play a little golf or stroll with a dog.

The third possibility is that coronary thrombosis is due to an insidous poison present in the modern environment, and at present the prime suspect is carbon monoxide. This gas is released into the atmosphere from vehicle exhausts, and is also an ingredient of smoke from tobacco, marihuana and even herbal mixtures. The evidence is reviewed in detail elsewhere in this book but there are persuasive arguments that cigarette smoking is one of the most important causes of the epidemic of heart disease. Another environmental factor that is still a mystery is the effect of soft water (p. 53). Inhabitants of areas of the country with soft water have about twice the mortality rate from heart disease found in hard-water areas. As yet this difference is quite unexplained.

Most health authorities now accept that all these factors – and others – combine together to account for the high incidence of coronary thrombosis. Individuals with diabetes, high blood pressure and other diseases are known to have an increased risk of heart disease, and the purpose of most health-screening programmes is the identification of persons with multiple risk factors. Someone with high blood pressure, overweight, who ate a high fat diet and smoked forty cigarettes daily, took no exercise and lived under great em otional stress would clearly be advised to try to eliminate at least some of these risk factors.

Stroke is a sudden event – a thrombosis, a haemorrhage or an embolism – affecting the blood-vessels of the brain, causing loss of function which may be temporary or permanent. While strokes cause about as many deaths each year as coronary thrombosis they have attracted less research, probably because their main effect on mortality is after the age of sixty. Between forty-one and sixty, deaths from coronary thrombosis are three times as numerous as those due to stroke; between sixty and eighty they are roughly equal; and over the age of eighty strokes cause nearly twice as many deaths as heart disease.

Yet these two great killers are manifestations of one disease, atherosclerosis, which narrows the blood-vessels in all parts of the body. It just happens that this narrowing seems less well tolerated by the coronary arteries supplying blood to the heart than by the blood-vessels supplying the brain. Over 300 years ago the English anatomist Thomas Willis showed that there is a circle of arteries at the base of the brain: four main arteries carry blood to it from the heart and eight branches lead from it to all parts of the brain. Blockage of part of this system can be compensated by increase in blood-flow elsewhere. Furthermore, doctors are still amazed by the power of recovery of the brain: some months after an incapacitating stroke, mental and physical function may be back to near normal.

However, strokes are dangerous events: only half the 100,000 persons who have a stroke each year in Britain are alive one month later. Little is known of the factors that precipitate a stroke rather than a coronary thrombosis in someone with atherosclerosis. The risk factors seem the same: high blood pressure, diabetes, too much cholesterol in the blood, overweight and cigarette smoking. Even the personality factors seem the same.

The most recently recognized risk factor is the contraceptive pill. Oral contraceptives affect the balance of clotting agents in the blood, and so predispose to thrombosis in both veins and arteries. Women on the pill, therefore, have an increased risk of both stroke and coronary thrombosis – and indeed the pill seems to be a factor in about a third of the very rare deaths from these causes in women aged less than forty-five years. These circumstances emphasize the close similarity of stroke and heart attack – and indeed anyone who solves the problem of coronary disease will be well on the way to reducing mortality from stroke, too.

CHEST DISEASE

Bronchitis, asthma and related chest diseases account for nearly as many deaths as stroke and heart disease; but many of these deaths are in the elderly and represent a way of dying rather than a cause of death. Pneumonia, indeed, used to be called the 'old man's friend' since it eased so many out of the world quietly, fairly quickly, and without much pain or discomfort. Too many people still die of bronchitis in middle age, however; at every age from forty onwards it causes more deaths than lung cancer.

As with so many other diseases, susceptibility to chest disease seems to depend just as much on genetic makeup as on environment and outside influences. 'Chestiness', like diabetes or short sight, runs in families; but this inborn susceptibility has been shown to be important more clearly for asthma and tuberculosis than for bronchitis. By far the most important cause of bronchitis is atmospheric pollution (p. 189). As the filthy air of industrial cities has been cleaned so has the incidence of bronchitis fallen; and, more important, the rate of progression of the disease has slowed. Even more important, however, is the role of personal pollution by tobacco smoking (p. 243).

BREAST CANCER

Cancer of all kinds is the third great killer in middle and old age. In contrast to heart disease and stroke, however, medical scientists are achieving real successes in identifying the causes of cancer and sometimes in eliminating them. Occupational tumours such as bladder cancer in rubber workers, nasal cancer in wood workers, skin cancer in tar workers, and chest cancer in asbestos workers (p. 165) can be and are being prevented by modifications to industrial processes. Prevention of lung cancer due to cigarette smoking is less easy, since banning smoking is argued to be an unjustifiable interference with individual freedom, and persuasion has so far had little effect.

Breast cancer is perhaps the most feared of the major cancers. It is the commonest form of the disease in women: each year there are more than 30,000 operations for breast cancer in Britain and over 10,000 deaths. Despite research efforts, little is known of the cause of breast cancer, but its preponderance in women (though a few cases do occur in men) suggests that hormonal factors have a major role. There is a sharp increase in the incidence of the disease in the years preceding the menopause, when changes in hormone balance occur, and the condition is more common in women with early puberty and a late menopause. Early pregnancy seems to protect against the disease in some way — a woman who has her first child before the age of eighteen has only a quarter of the risk of breast cancer of a woman who has no children or whose first pregnancy is delayed until the age of thirty-five. It seems that pregnancy is the crucial factor; whether or not the baby is breast-fed seems irrelevant. Since pregnancy has a protective effect, not surprisingly women who take oral contraceptives (which to some extent reproduce the hormonal state of pregnancy) certainly have no increased risk of breast cancer and may have a lower risk. This hormonal dependence is of vital importance to surgeons treating women with breast cancer. The best chance of cure is given by early surgical removal of the tumour, sometimes backed up by treatment with anti-cancer drugs. Nevertheless, in those cases in which metastases are found in the bones or liver, hormone treatment may be highly effective, and the optimum choice of hormones may be found by studying their effect on laboratory growth of cancer cells taken from the individual woman's tumour.

Hormones are not the only influence on breast cancer, however; almost certainly there are external factors too. This is most strikingly shown by studies of the disease in Japanese women. Some of the common cancers found in Western society, including breast cancer, are rare in Japan; but when Japanese emigrate to the USA they soon begin to show an American pattern of cancer. Women born in America of pure Japanese parentage have much the same incidence of breast cancer as that in white Americans. At present the view of cancer specialists is that some unknown environmental factor found in Japan protects against breast cancer, rather than there being a cancer-causing environmental poison in the USA.

Hormones are also known to have a strong influence on cancer of the uterus, and there has been much medical anxiety about the effects of long-term therapy with sex hormones. So far the balance of evidence has suggested that oral contraceptives do not increase the risk of cancer of the uterus. The same cannot be said for hormone replacement therapy – the use of long-term oestrogen therapy to maintain the body in a pre-menopausal state and so to slow the effects of ageing on the bones, skin, and possibly the mental state. This form of treatment, very widely prescribed in North America, was shown in 1975 to be associated with an increased risk of endometrial carcinoma (cancer of the lining of the uterus). In Britain hormone replacement therapy is less widely prescribed, and many gynaecologists prefer to prescribe an alternative regimen which mimics the contraceptive pill and contains a progestogen as well as an oestrogen. This combination, given for only three weeks a month, is claimed to protect against uterine cancer, but long-term trials have not yet been completed.

LUNG CANCER

If the cause of breast cancer remains a mystery there is no such doubt about lung cancer, which accounts for the deaths each year in Britain of 25,000 men and 5,000 women. The role of tobacco in the causation of lung cancer has been unravelled to the satisfaction of all but a few sceptics (p. 256), but other aspects are still puzzling.

Undoubtedly tobacco may sometimes act in conjunction with other environmental agents in greatly increasing the incidence of lung cancer. Asbestos, for example, is one industrial cause of lung cancer: it seems that asbestos workers who smoke have ninety times the risk in non-smokers of developing lung cancer and dying from it. A similar relationship seems to exist with other occupational causes of lung cancer such as gold mining and carbonization of coal. These relationships have raised the question of whether there might be an unidentified co-agent working with tobacco in causing non-industrial lung cancer. Such a theory became popular when evidence was first published showing that in many parts of the world the death rate from lung cancer is higher in towns and cities than in the countryside. Could atmospheric pollution, possibly due to motor-vehicle exhausts, be the critical factor?

Disproving such a hypothesis is always difficult. However, in its detailed examination of smoking in 1970 the Royal College of Physicians concluded that the evidence against the importance of community air pollution as a cause of lung cancer was stronger than the evidence for it. The difference between lung cancer rates in town and country is greatest in Sweden, Norway and Denmark – countries with the lowest levels of urban air pollution. However, emigrants from cities in Britain to the USA, South Africa, New Zealand and Australia seem to carry their susceptibility to lung cancer with them, suggesting an environmental factor operating early in life. Confirmation of this possibility is given by the low lung-cancer rate in Norwegian migrants to the USA.

At present the view of the World Health Organization is that while there is an undoubted increased risk of lung cancer for town-dwellers the cause remains unknown, but is unlikely to be simple atmospheric pollution. Cigarette smoking remains the only identified factor of any importance.

STOMACH AND BOWEL CANCER

Stomach cancer kills 15,000 people each year in Britain, putting it second only to the lung in the league table of cancer deaths; yet very little is known about its cause. Both in Britain and in the USA the condition is apparently becoming less common; but again the reasons are unknown. Stomach cancer is more prevalent in the poorer social classes; it occurs more often in men than women and slightly more often in those with blood group A; and there are appreciable racial variations. There is, for example, evidence that the disease is slightly more common in the Welsh than the English, while Japanese have more stomach cancer than any other developed nation. As yet, however, no one has been able to show a clear link between stomach cancer and any type of food, drink or occupation.

Bowel cancer is almost as big an enigma, with an added difficulty: cancers of the twenty-odd feet of small intestine are extremely rare, while in the six feet of large intestine they are very common. Oddly enough, international variations of bowel cancer contrast sharply with those of stomach cancer; growths of the intestines are common in the USA and relatively rare in Japan. As with stomach cancer, no environmental cause of the disease has been identified with any certainty, but some medical authorities believe that the modern Western diet may be responsible. Compared with our ancestors' diet, current Western food contains far less indigestible vegetable fibre and far more sugar (p. 49). These changes have two effects: the contents of the intestine move more slowly, and the bacteria in the bowel have changed to different species. Could it be that the new bacteria produce poisons, or toxins, which are kept in contact with the lining of the bowel as a result of its sluggish movement, and that these toxins are the cause of bowel cancer? As yet such a theory has no hard evidence to support it, but it fits in with a little of the evidence.

GENITAL CANCER

Too much publicity may have been given to reports linking genital cancer in both men and women to sexual activity. Certainly there is some evidence that cancer of the cervix in women and of the prostate in men are found more often in those who started sexual activity young and changed partners frequently. Most of the data relate to women, but there is also some evidence that promiscuous behaviour by husbands may increase the risk of cervical cancer in their wives. Wives of fishermen and boatmen have twenty times the risk of cervical cancer found in the wives of clergymen. Nevertheless, the most important factor in determining mortality seems to be social class – probably linked with the reluctance of working women to seek medical treatment early on. Cervical cancer is substantially less common than breast cancer: diagnosed early it can be treated effectively; and at present the death rate is steadily falling. It seems to be one of the cancers that could be brought under control with the knowledge we already possess.

CONCLUSION

Perhaps the most remarkable inference that can be drawn from this survey of the known causes of disease, disability and death is man's resilience. Many miners can and do spend their lives at the coal-face without developing pneumoconiosis; a few life-long cigarette smokers play tennis in their seventies; some overweight businessmen spend their lives in an alcoholic haze without developing cirrhosis of the liver. Everyone has a friend or relation who has ignored all the medical rules and yet remained healthy until well past retirement.

For most of us, however, the lessons are clear. The big dangers to health come from eating too much (and especially too much carbohydrate); drinking alcohol to excess; smoking cigarettes; and driving a car while not wearing a seat-belt. Avoid those hazards, and you should live to collect your pension – and be fit enough to enjoy it.

INDEX

Abnormalities, birth, 13, 219,
278, 288, 289; and regional
variation, 278, 280; and soft
water, 53
Abortion, 259, 260, 290, 291
Accidents, in childhood, 295; in
coal-miners, 142, 143; and
deep-sea diving, 148; and
drug-addicts, 227; and farm
animals, 170; fatal, and
trawlermen, 149; industrial,
152, 213; and injuries, 296;
and obesity, 38; tractor, 170;
and trawlermen, 149, 150
Accidents, road, 27, 137, 265,
296; and alcoholism, 213, 219,
295–6
Achondroplasia, 281
Acheson, Professor Donald, 141
Acid, sulphuric, 192
Action on Smoking and Health
(ASH), 233
Acute lead poisoning, 197
Addiction, to Benzedrine, cocaine
Dexedrine, glue, heroin,
morphine, psychedelic drugs,
224–9; and broken homes, 226;
to chlorodyne, 98; drug, 31,
133, 224–9; to purgatives, 94;
to smoking, 223, 237
Additives, food, 72
Adrenaline, 234
Aerosol deodorants, 182
Aflatoxins, 69
Agar, 94
Agent, anti-knock, 195
Air, compressed, illness, 162

Aircraft noise, 199, 200
Alcohol, 87, 212–19; and aspirin,
87; and the brain, 213, 217;
and driving, 219, 296; and
health, 217; and punch-
drunkenness, 114
Alcoholic cardiomyopathy,
218
Alcoholism, 14, 212; and
analgesic abusers 91; and
effect on unborn child, 287;
and parasuicide, 32; prevalence
of, according to county, 212,
213; and vitamin B deficiency,
56, 219
Alconyidium gelatinosum, 152
Allergic lung diseases, 164, 181
Allergy to sea chervil, 152
Alzheimer's disease, 93
Amenorrhoea, 267, 268
Aminopterin, 290
Amoeba, 77, 96
Amotivational syndrome, 223
Amphetamine, 222, 225, 231
Anabolic steroids, 229, 230
Anaemia, 56, 87, 197, 230
Anaemia, and anabolic steroids,
230; and aspirin, 87; and lead,
197; pernicious, in vegans, 56;
and pregnancy, 283
Anaesthetic gases, effect on an
unborn baby, 288
Analgesic nephropathy, 90
Analgesics, 86
Anderson, Dr John, 40
Anencephaly, 53, 280
Anger, fear, irritation and
coronary heart disease, 299

INDEX

MORE ABOUT PENGUINS
AND PELICANS

Penguinews, which appears every month, contains details of all the new books issued by Penguins as they are published. From time to time it is supplemented by *Penguins in Print*, which is our complete list of almost 5,000 titles.

A specimen copy of *Penguinews* will be sent to you free on request. Please write to Dept EP, Penguin Books Ltd, Harmondsworth, Middlesex, for your copy.

In the U.S.A.: For a complete list of books available from Penguins in the United States write to Dept CS, Penguin Books, 625 Madison Avenue, New York, New York 10022.

In Canada: For a complete list of books available from Penguins in Canada write to Penguin Books Canada Ltd, 41 Steelcase Road West, Markham, Ontario.

SOME BOOKS ON BIOLOGY AND
NATURAL HISTORY PUBLISHED IN
PENGUINS

Nature Through the Seasons *Richard Adams and
Max Hooper*

Silent Spring *Rachel Carson*

The Origin of Species *Charles Darwin (Ed. J. W. Burrow)*

A Dictionary of Biology

A Dictionary of Science

The Growth of Plants *C. E. Fogg*

Human Populations *David Hay*

Grasses *C. E. Hubbard*

Apes, Men, and Language *Eugene Linden*

The Soul of the Ape *Eugene Marais*

The Soul of the White Ant *Eugene Marais*

Microbes and Man *John Postgate*

Parasites *A. J. Probert*

Ornithology: An Introduction *Austin L. Rand*

Man and the Vertebrates (2 volumes) *Alfred Sherwood
Romer*

The Chemistry of Life *Steven Rose*

The Conscious Brain *Steven Rose*

Season on the Plain *Franklin Russell*

The Year of the Seal *Victor Scheffer*

The Year of the Whale *Victor Scheffer*

Space Biology *G. F. Stoneman*

Hormones and the Body *A. Stuart Mason*

MAGICAL MEDICINE

A Nigerian Case-Study

Una Maclean

The real value of African medicine, as the author points out in this Pelican, lies not in its materials but in the methods and concepts which underlie their use. It is characterized by its ability to supply meaningful answers to questions which are relevant to patient and practitioner alike.

Basing her study on the town of Ibadan in Nigeria, Una Maclean describes the failure of modern European medicine to replace the herbalist and diviner, and shows how these two types of medicine continue to exist side by side. And, to further illustrate her argument, she analyses the results of her survey of native healers and child-rearing mothers.

A fascinating study in itself, *Magical Medicine* also raises the question of whether, by concentrating on accurate diagnosis and cure, Western medicine has lost sight of the necessity of treating the patient as a whole man.

'A wise and careful study' – *The Times Literary Supplement*

HORMONES AND THE BODY

A. Stuart Mason

Hormones are the very stuff of life. Secreted by the endocrine glands, floating in the bloodstream, they regulate chemically almost every bodily process – be it growth, lactation or simply the reduction of blood sugar levels.

The role of adrenalin, the way 'the Pill' works, the nature of diabetes and the problems of fatness and thinness are all explained in Doctor Mason's readable and comprehensive book. Originally published in Pelicans under the title *Health and Hormones*, it has now been brought thoroughly up to date and expanded. Doctor Mason explains the nature of hormones and the structure of the endocrine system as a whole, chapter by chapter, from the pituitary to the pancreas, making clear the significance of each for bodily health.

MEDICINE AND MAN

Noël Poynter

Medicine has had a momentous effect on man. Our expectation of life and our attitude towards death, the structure of societies and the bonds between nations have been radically changed since man became able to fight disease.

Inevitably ethics, politics, philosophy, religion and education have not only left their mark on the history of medicine but have themselves been altered in their turn.

Medicine and Man is a fascinating study of these interactions. Its author, Dr Noël Poynter, an eminent medical historian, offers not a narrative history but, as one critic wrote, 'a splendid survey of contemporary social and intellectual problems of medicine'. The subjects include the question of abortion and population control, the treatment of the aged and infirm, the historical forces at work on the development of medical care in England, and the central role of medicine both in today's society and in the world of tomorrow.